WADING INTO CHAOS

BOB HOLDSWORTH

WADING INTO CHAOS:

INSIDE THE LIFE OF A PARAMEDIC

Advantage.

Published by Advantage, Charleston, South Carolina.
Member of Advantage Media Group.

ADVANTAGE is a registered trademark and the Advantage colophon is a trademark of Advantage Media Group, Inc.

Printed in the United States of America.

ISBN: 978-159932-356-5
LCCN: 2012955488

This publication is designed to provide accurate and authoritative information in regard to the subject matter covered. It is sold with the understanding that the publisher is not engaged in rendering legal, accounting, or other professional services. If legal advice or other expert assistance is required, the services of a competent professional person should be sought.

Advantage Media Group is proud to be a part of the Tree Neutral® program. Tree Neutral offsets the number of trees consumed in the production and printing of this book by taking proactive steps such as planting trees in direct proportion to the number of trees used to print books. To learn more about Tree Neutral, please visit **www.treeneutral.com**. To learn more about Advantage's commitment to being a responsible steward of the environment, please visit **www.advantagefamily.com/green**

Advantage Media Group is a leading publisher of business, motivation, and self-help authors. Do you have a manuscript or book idea that you would like to have considered for publication? Please visit **www.advantagefamily.com** or call **1.866.775.1696**

DEDICATION

Thank you to all of my ambulance partners past, present, and future, and to all who provide emergency medical services (EMS) around the world; I'm proud to be a part of the fraternity.

To the most important partner I've ever had in life: Jennifer, thank you for putting up with me, for loving me even when I made it difficult, for supporting me and for showing me that there is a whole lot more to life.

You're my best friend…all my love…all my life.

TABLE OF CONTENTS

AUTHOR'S NOTE

My name is Bob Holdsworth. I've worked in emergency medicine for thirty-three years, first as a volunteer firefighter and emergency medical technician (EMT), and then as a paramedic from 1986 to the present. I also spent four and a half years in prison—as a corrections officer and medic in a maximum-security jail.

Over that span of time, I've been directly involved with the care of more than 20,000 patients, and that is a conservative estimate. I've kept a count of certain types of calls simply out of morbid curiosity.

I give you the following statistics not to brag in any way, but just to give you a glimpse into the scope of cases that I've been involved with and that has shaped my perspective of the world, and my ability and desire to write about it.

Cardiac Arrests	863	(victims aged 3 months–101)
Shootings	534	(victims aged 5–77)
Stabbings	678	(including being stabbed on the job)
Hangings	97	(victims aged 14–82)
Fatal Motor Vehicle Crashes	236	(victims aged 3–95)
Fire-related deaths	29	(victims aged 2–89)
Fatal suicides, nonhanging	287	(victims aged 10–90)

The following stories are all based in reality, meaning the calls actually took place. I have taken some writer's license within these boundaries: names have been changed either to limit further pain for victims and families or because partners have opted not to have their names published.

I am proud to be involved in this profession, to have been given the opportunity to impact the lives of others, and to now be able to share some of those interactions with you.

As you read these vignettes, I want you to place yourself at the scene; try to visualize it, see the sights, smell the smells, experience the emotion, and briefly sample what emergency medical service personnel all over the world experience every day, taking risks for all of us by wading into chaos.

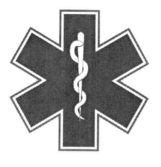

CHAPTER 1

CURIOSITY: THE BEGINNING

CURIOSITY: THE BEGINNING

It's amazing how a seemingly insignificant turn in the road can change the direction of your life, and wind up taking you places you never expected to go, for instance, into an ambulance.

My first time away from home came in 1977 when I went to the University of Hartford. I was looking for some folks to hang out with and a way to fit in. One of the guys on my dorm floor was involved with emergency services; he was an "ambulance driver."

Because of the maze of dorms and other buildings on campus, ambulance crews got lost trying to find patients, causing potentially lethal delays. We talked about it and decided that, with the approval of campus security, we'd form a first-responder group to help reduce the delays. So, we all took a CPR and first-aid course. We were harassed for it by the drunken students around campus, but we started responding within the dorms. We'd arrive, start taking care of people, and then direct the ambulance to wherever the injured person was. Typically, we worked Friday and Saturday nights, dealing with kids who were too drunk to stand and fell down and banged their heads, with the occasional seizure or overdose, and with guys who got in a fight and ended up with a bloody lip, nothing too extreme, a little bit of blood here and there. We'd put a bandage on the wound and wait for the ambulance to show up. To my surprise, I really enjoyed it.

My new-found friend, Blair, worked on the ambulance in Hartford. He responded to the university when he was working, and we'd turn the patient over to him. One night, when we were having a beer, I asked him, "What happens after you guys come in and put them on the stretcher and take off? What's the rest of the story?"

He said, "Well, why don't you come ride?"

Why not?

"Okay. Make it happen."

A couple of Friday nights later, Blair called me. "We'll pick you up at four, and we're on until midnight. If it gets busy, we're on past midnight, so plan for that."

Friday came, and he and his partner picked me up in the ambulance. I got into the truck, and he said, "Pull the medical box up and sit on that." So I perched in between them in a narrow cut-through between the cab and the patient compartment. This was long before anybody cared about seat belts. Sounds of radio traffic, codes, numbers, and all kinds of conversation filled the cabin. I was talking to him and getting acclimated to the whole thing when without warning we're rocketing down the street with the lights and siren on.

"What the hell just happened? I didn't hear anything."

"We're going to a motor vehicle accident. It just came over the radio."

How could that be? The radio is six inches from my knee and I didn't hear a thing.

"You'll catch on."

We got to the scene, and he told me, "Stay out of the way, but hand me stuff when I tell you to."

Everything was moving fast; collars, and backboards, oxygen, radio reports to the hospital—a million and one things were going on at the same time, all compacted into fourteen minutes from the time the lights and sirens were turned on to arrival at the emergency department. Watching Blair work, I realized I didn't know him at all. I knew the crazy off-duty side, because we drank and goofed off together. But this—this I hadn't seen.

Crap. He can be serious. Who knew?

I was awed, watching the organization that went into it, the choreography, if you will, of arriving, placing the vehicle in a safe spot, getting out, watching traffic, taking care of the patient, becoming an advocate for that patient—their best friend—all in literally seconds. These are people who are upset and confused and hurt, often with panicked family members watching at the scene too. You've got to wade into the middle of the chaos and quickly and calmly get things under control. Your whole demeanor has to send the message: "I'm here. It's okay. Relax. We've got this under control. We'll take care of it. We'll take care of *you.*"

All I could think as I watched them work was, *This is really cool.* I'd been in the restaurant business since I was fifteen, serving customers, cooking up hamburgers and serving ice cream. I had worked my way to management by the time I was eighteen and had assumed that that would be my professional life. Suddenly, at nineteen, that didn't seem nearly as attractive.

I've always been up for a challenge. My dad and his father were both in bank management in Boston. My other grandfather was probably one of the best-known jewelry repair guys in Boston. They taught me how to manage things, lead people, and fix things, and they gave me a strong work ethic: I was always taught that if something needed to get done, just get it done. Seeing this all come together on the streets, with the stakes raised higher, made the job that much more appealing. I knew I simply had to get involved; I had to do this job!

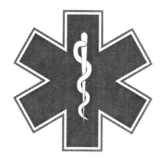

CHAPTER 2

CLASSES, CLASSES, CLASSES

CLASSES, CLASSES, CLASSES

My wife accuses me of having undiagnosed attention deficit disorder, and I don't know if I was bored with what I was doing, or if the bright shiny object of the ambulance with the flashing lights was my inner toddler's fire-truck-loving dream come true, but when the night was over, my first question was, "Where do I find myself an EMT class?" I had already decided that I was dropping out of college at the end of the semester, having accepted a management position with a restaurant chain. I was living in Farmington, so I called the fire department and was told, "Yeah, if you come join, we'll get you into training and we'll pay for your EMT class."

Sold!

When people ask me how I ended up doing what I do, I always say I lost a bet, because when I told my friend Blair that I was going to take the EMT class, he said I'd never go through with it all, and I said, "Okay, I'll prove you wrong."

So, for the next six months, I went to fire school on weekends, took two EMT classes a week at night, and worked full-time managing a Friendly's restaurant. Six crazy, overcommitted months of broken bones, bleeding, shock, CPR: "How did you want your burger?"; Okay, I've got to ladder the building and I've got to tie an overhand knot into the harness because I'm going to slide down the side of the building now; "Oh, I'm opening tomorrow? Okay. How'd you want your eggs?"

For six months I didn't know whether I was coming or going. I had the red book for fire, the orange book for EMS, and the blue book for ordering ice cream for the store. I'd get up, thinking, *Where am I and what uniform am I supposed to wear today?* People would ask, "Hey, you want to go drinking?"

"No. I've got fire school in the morning."

"You've got what?"

"Hey, you want to go out to dinner?"

"No. I've got an EMT practical tonight. I'm learning splinting tonight."

"Okay, well, we'll have a beer for you."

"Okay. That'd be great. Have at it."

I had the scanner going at night listening for "the big one."

After three months, when I had finished a certain number of courses, I was deemed eligible to respond to fire calls, and I put a blue light and fire gear in my car. Now I'm either going out the door in a Friendly's uniform, or it's two in the morning and I'm running out the door, waking up my roommates, because there's a smoke alarm activation somewhere in town, and I've got to run to the firehouse. My roommates thought I was insane.

"What are you *doing*, dude?"

"I don't know, but I'm having fun."

"Well, can you turn the freaking scanner down because you're keeping us awake?"

"Nope. I have to listen to other noises coming from your room. Cope."

I still didn't know what I wanted from all this, but I knew I wanted something. When I started, my intent was to join the fire department, get my EMT certification, then join an ambulance service, and pull a shift a week on Friday night or on the weekend. I was going to keep working for the restaurant because it was a good job, and it paid well.

When I finally graduated from my EMT class and the fire academy, I was a member of the Oakland Gardens Fire Department in Farmington, CT, a one-engine station right near my house. It was a relatively quiet station; we had a few fires, some medical calls—a good place to get my feet wet. But it wasn't busy enough for me; I was eager to put my new skills to a tougher test.

A paramedic unit was stationed at the UCONN Health Center down the street, and I connected with two guys there: Carmen and Jerry. I asked them if I could ride with them because now that I'd seen what the ambulance crews did, I wondered what the hell the paramedics did. The show *Emergency!* was on TV and we all watched it. These guys from UCONN were in a nontransport, squad-type vehicle, just like the show's heroes, Johnny and Roy. I wanted to go ride.

Once again, I found myself sitting on the drug box in between the seats as we raced to calls. It was starting to feel like my natural spot. I learned from watching them that there was a lot more to EMS that what I'd just learned in EMT class.

As soon as I got my EMT certification, I joined the West Hartford Volunteer Ambulance service. The first time I drove up, I saw the organization's truck, an old Dodge van ambulance, which I discovered was notorious for not starting. We'd respond to a call and the starter would go *rurrh-rurrh-rurrh*. The standard answer was, "Okay. Let's jump it and go."

I had seen the units of the Professional Ambulance Service. They were red, white, and blue, and modern looking, and here's this Dodge ambulance with an orange stripe, two little red bubble lights, and a siren in between, with curtains on the back windows. Interesting.

The "office" was on the second floor of a small, combination-retail-apartment-type building, so I went up and announced, "I'd like to join." They took my application and said they'd call. A couple of days later, they did.

"Hey, this is Bruce. You've been accepted as a probationary member. We'd like you to come down and meet some folks and do some orientation. How's Friday?"

Friday comes and this time I take a better look around their headquarters, which consisted of a couple of couches, a TV, a desk with a map of the town over it and a single microphone on it, and the radio; kind of drab surroundings.

"Where do the calls come from? Do you guys answer 9-1-1 here?"

"No. The West Hartford Police dispatchers answer the calls and then they call us or the other service, Professional."

Bruce showed me around and introduced me to a couple of people. They were all sitting around watching TV and drinking coffee.

Bruce said, "You and I are going to be working together a lot until I get you through orientation, okay?"

He was a slightly built guy, about my age, who'd lived in West Hartford all his life and told me he knew the town like the back of his hand.

"Okay."

His partner Willie was an older guy, a professional truck driver who came down to ride the ambulance. He was our maintenance guy too. He'd been around for a long time, doing ambulance calls since before there was such a thing as an EMT certification.

"Okay. Well, this is cool. I'll ride with you guys. How many calls do you get?"

"Not a lot."

So, I spent the night with them. Nothing.

At about 11:00 pm they announced, "We're going to go out and get some coffee."

We walked over to the coffee shop, which was around the corner, close enough for us to run back to the ambulance if we needed to. We didn't take the ambulance with us, because we might not have gotten our parking space back.

I worked a lot of Friday nights, and we would go over to the coffee shop and chat for hours, waiting for something to happen. Every once in a while, because it was so quiet, somebody would do a radio check with the police department just to see if the thing was working. We'd watch Professional Ambulance Service go screaming by us, and we'd call the police department to make sure our radio was working, and they'd tell us, "Yep, it's working."

I discovered that for the serious accidents, they just automatically bypassed the volunteers and went to Professional's crews. The dispatchers couldn't be bothered to try to keep track of who was next up in the rotation system and who wasn't, even though we'd call them and tell them we were in service. It was easier for them to speed dial the other guys and send them.

One night Bruce decided that he was going to take me out to show me around West Hartford so I could learn some of the main roads. He was showing me how to use the ambulance and how the lights worked, making sure I could back up without hitting anything in a parking lot when we finally got a call—a difficulty-breathing call—on the other side of West Hartford. I was driving.

"I'll take care of the map," Bruce told me. "Go down three streets, take a right on Farmington."

So, I took a right on Farmington, and as I did that, I looked over and watched him turn the map to the right.

I kept driving.

"Oh, okay. Go down here, four streets, and at the next traffic light, take a left."

"Okay."

I started making a left turn. He turned the map to the left.

What in the hell is he doing?

"It's like four streets down on the right, and then there's a little cul-de-sac we've got to find."

So, I kept driving, turned right, and he turned the map to the right *again*.

I finally stopped the truck. "What the hell are you doing? Why are you turning the map every time I turn the truck?"

"I don't know. It's just how I learned to do it. I'll teach you how to do it later."

"No. No, you won't. Thanks for the map reading class. I'm good. We're here, by the way."

We'd arrived at a small cape-style home, and inside we found a little old grey-haired lady sitting at her kitchen table in her nightgown. Her house smelled like a little old lady's house: a mixture of stale food, liniment, dust, and—ah yes—cats.

How many cats do you have? There's either a crap load of cats, you haven't cleaned the litter box in a while, or you have a mountain lion in the next room, and it's hot—very hot!

She's got her cross word puzzle out. She's got her home oxygen device on. She had a cup of coffee and a cigarette going. It was about eighty-eight degrees in the house, yet it was a nice sixty-degree evening outside. Now *I was* having trouble breathing because of the ammonia stink from the cat box. My eyes watered. It was hot. We needed to go *now*.

"Do you always have trouble breathing?"

"No. Not always. Sometimes."

"Does it happen a lot when it gets really hot and you're smoking?"

"Sometimes."

"Okay. Maybe we might want to open a window?"

"Oh, no, no, no. I get too cold too quickly."

"Okay. What would you like to do?"

"Oh, I want to go to the hospital. I called my doctor and he said that I should go get checked out."

She wheezed a little bit.

"Are you having trouble breathing?"

"Well, I used my inhaler and it's not working."

"How many times did you use your inhaler?"

"Six."

Typically, you use an inhaler once, maybe twice, because if you use it more often, it begins to work the opposite of how it's supposed to, and it also can raise your heart rate. The last thing you want to do to people who have cardiac and respiratory problems is raise their heart rate, make an irregular heartbeat worse, or raise blood pressure. Her heart rate was 120. She was breathing too quickly, not getting enough oxygen, and she had emphysema, a result of smoking for forty years. And she was still smoking.

"Why don't we put the cigarette out? We're going to switch you over to our oxygen bottle, and we'll put you in the stair chair," which is a carrying device, a chair with wheels and handles. "We'll cover you with the sheet; we'll strap you in; and we'll take you down to the hospital and get you checked."

We got her down the stairs and out of the ammonia-laden, overheated room to the beautiful evening outside. Miraculously she began to breathe more easily.

"Oh, I feel better already."

"Yeah, me too."

Bruce drove us to St. Francis Hospital, and all the way there she was able to breathe much better. She talked about her grandchildren, her cat, Buttons, what a wonderful day it was and how nice we were, and she kept holding my hand. I realized, for all the stupidity, the drunks, the blood, and other disasters we ran across, making a difference in this lady's life for twenty minutes was a really cool deal.

Over the years, calls like this one act as a reset button. Every call that challenges you, that makes you think, that gives you nightmares, leaves a mark. The longer you're in EMS, the more marks. They all return at some point to haunt you, and then there's the one little-old-lady call that really didn't tax your skills too much. She needed a little oxygen. She needed some fresh air. She needed a little bit of medicine after the overuse of her inhaler to control her wheezing. But really, she just wanted to talk about her grandkids. She just wanted to have her blood pressure checked. She just wanted to tell us what nice young men we were and to hold my hand on the way to the hospital. It resets your humanity gyroscope so that you can go on.

Her name was Grace. She was a devout Catholic and told me all about her mother. Her mother named her Grace because her favorite song was "Amazing Grace." She was all alone now; it was just her and Buttons.

I said, "Well, I'll give you a piece of advice. You should stop smoking."

"Yes, yes, I know."

"You also should never use your inhaler that much, and you really should move Buttons's litter box someplace because I think the ammonia's causing you trouble."

"Oh, okay. That's a good idea. Maybe I'll clean it once every week."

"Yep, that's a good idea. You should do that."

It had been nearly a year since I'd started down this EMS journey, and it was starting to feel more and more like what I should be doing with my life, not something to do in my spare time. I was having more fun doing my unpaid stuff than I was managing a restaurant. The West Hartford Ambulance service wasn't all that busy and I wanted more action, so I applied to Professional Ambulance Service, which was the ambulance service where I'd ridden with Blair. They hired me on the spot. At that time, if you had an EMT card and could fog a mirror, you were hired.

On my first night on the job, I went in for my orientation. As I walked through the door—and it was a really busy night—they looked at my new shirt and freshly sewn-on EMT patch. "You're an EMT?"

"Yeah, I'm here for my orientation."

"You're going to get it. Go with Lynn."

"Go with Lynn where?"

"You've got a call."

So much for orientation. We went out to the truck and got in. She said, "Put your seat belt on. Let's go."

"Where are we going?"

She very calmly said, "Oh, we have a shooting." She wheeled the ambulance all the way through town toward the north end of Hartford.

On the way, she said, "Pay attention to the scene. Pay attention to everybody around you. It is very important that you learn where the guy with the gun or the guy with the knife is, before you turn your back on anybody."

Okay, city lesson number one.

Hartford was a tough town: lots of gangs, lots of drugs, lots of crime. Cops called the north end of Hartford the Knife and Gun Club and the south end of Hartford the Knife and Pipe Club, because the north end tended to produce more shootings and stabbings and the south end tended to have more stabbings and beatings. It was not at all uncommon for every ambulance on the road to catch a shooting or a stabbing on every shift. I was a kid from the suburbs, so this was all new to me.

We pulled up in front of this house, a typical inner city house with two stories, two porches, and a streetlight over it. There were twenty or thirty people on the front lawn, so I knew there'd been a party. When we and the cops arrived, they all started to drift away. Nobody wanted to be involved. After we stepped out of the truck, Lynn looked at everybody and asked, "Where is the person?"

A couple of people pointed at the first-floor door. We went in to see, writhing on the kitchen floor, a young black guy, semiconscious, holding his abdomen, moaning. A young lady was leaning over him, saying, "You'll be okay. You'll be okay."

I remembered to ask, "Where's the guy that shot him?" She told me he'd left. Lynn already had a bandage out and on the wound, assessing it.

"Okay, we've got to roll him over and look to see if there's an exit wound."

Right. I knew that.

Always look for the exit wound in a gunshot case.

So, we rolled him over; no exit wound. Suddenly, it was a more serious call.

Typically when a gunshot wound has an exit, you can determine the trajectory of the bullet. When there's no exit wound, it means the bullet could be anywhere and could have bounced around and done lots of damage. So, all of a sudden, it goes from, "All right, the victim's shot in the abdomen," which is critical but not life threatening, to hypercritical because the bullet could have bounced off a rib and then into the heart or lung.

In this case, the victim had been shot in the abdomen, but I didn't know where the bullet was. We had to move.

The lady was freaking out. Lynn told her, "I've got it. We're taking care of him. We're going to move him in a minute, but I need to know for my own safety where the shooter is."

"If he comes back, I'll tell you."

Not comforting. Time to go.

Lynn looked at me. "Go get the backboard. We'll strap him down, and we'll take him out. Leave the stretcher at the stairs."

I reached into the ambulance, trying to remember how to make the bar work to unlock the stretcher, how to pull the stretcher out and get it to release so that the wheels come down and it won't be low to the ground, and I have to do this alone, in front of an interested audience of twenty-five people. It went very poorly. I could not figure out how to manage the eighty-pound stretcher. I barely got it out of the truck, and I couldn't get the wheels to drop. So, I had to wheel it completely down on the ground. I could feel everyone watching me. I took the straps off, unrolled the sheets so we had a place to put the backboard, and walked in with the backboard. "It's out there," I said.

We put the shooting victim on the board, strapped him down, and carried him out feet first, down the front steps. The way the stretcher was set up, we'd be putting the patient on the stretcher backward. Because I hadn't done this yet, I didn't know we were going to come out feet first. We had to go out and turn around to put the patient down so that the patient went in the ambulance correctly.

Lynn looked at the stretcher on the ground. "Why didn't you bring it up?"

"Because I couldn't figure out how to make it work."

We put him on the stretcher and strapped him in. Lynn grabbed the handle. "When I say 'three,' lift."

We raised it and now it looked like a stretcher. We wheeled him over to the ambulance, put him in, locked him in, and Lynn climbed in the back.

"What are you doing?"

"Drive me to the hospital."

"I have no idea how to operate this thing. I've never driven one like this. I've never taken a defensive driving course."

"See all those switches on the top row? Just hit them all. Turn the siren on and go."

"Okay, sure."

I hit 'em all. We had lights on that shouldn't have been on, all of the emergency lights, the siren was going, and we hadn't even pulled away from the house. In fact, I hadn't even put the ambulance in drive. The cop looked at me as if to ask what I was doing, because, unbeknownst to me, when you go into these situations, you're supposed to go in stealthily. And when you've got a shooting victim in an ambulance in front of twenty-five people who have been partying, and you turn on all the lights and the siren while you're still sitting there, parked, it attracts attention.

"Go!" Lynn yelled.

I put the vehicle in drive, and we go. Lynn took care of the patient and looked through the cut-through space (my old ride-along perch), giving me directions. "All right, next intersection. Take a left. Then, just go straight."

So, there was my first indoctrination into city EMS. I hadn't even punched in, and I'd already done a shooting.

This is pretty cool. I can do this.

When I accepted my first paid EMT job, Professional Ambulance was paying $3.75 an hour to do this work, so I knew I wasn't going to get rich.

But I really enjoyed it.

As it happened, about the same time, I was called in to my boss's office. I'd been doing well at the restaurant, and the company liked me, he explained. There was a new store opening up and they wanted me to take it on as the manager.

He said, "You've done a good job. Your numbers are good, and we know you can do it."

I knew it was a good career move for me: a big promotion with a big salary and profit sharing attached.

I didn't even have to think it over. "You know what? I don't want to. I know that I'm shooting myself in the foot income wise, but I just can't do it. I don't care how they want their burgers anymore. I really don't. I *do* care that I can be in somebody's house and stop the bleeding, control the scene, and get them to the emergency room alive. That's different than, 'I want my toast lightly browned and not buttered.' I'm actually going to resign."

My mother was not thrilled with this choice on a whole bunch of levels. She had not been thrilled when I announced that I was dropping out of college, and really not thrilled when I started going into burning buildings and riding on the backs of fire trucks, or cutting cars apart with the Jaws of Life. She wasn't happy that I was in the restaurant business because she didn't think that was going to be a long career for me, but now she was very, very unhappy that I was riding around on ambulances in the inner city. Then came the offer, and I never told her what the offer was. I just said, "They made me an offer. I'm not interested. I actually resigned."

At which point I got a motherly lecture. "So what are you going to do?"

"I'm going to go to work on the ambulance full-time."

"Well, what does that pay?"

"Less." I didn't tell her how much less.

"Huh. Really." My mother is not an overly expressive person, but her "Huh. Really." said volumes. I would start to tell her stories about what I had seen or done, and she did not want to hear them. If they involved shootings, car crashes, and people vomiting, she would immediately change the subject to, "So, who are you dating?" I didn't have much of an answer to that one.

She'd rather I'd taken this interest and gone to medical school, but quite frankly, I didn't like being inside all the time, and I didn't care for what I'd seen of hospital politics. It took a long time for her to finally realize that I was doing something good and making a living. I think she's okay with it now.

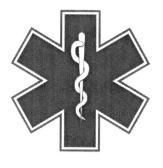

CHAPTER 3

SHOTS FIRED

SHOTS FIRED

In the early 1980s, the north end of Hartford was statistically one of the most violent areas in the country. It wasn't long after my orientation ride that I was assigned to the north end of Hartford, to a veteran EMT named Doug. He was a physically imposing guy and when he started telling a story, his voice and personality filled a room. Everybody would stop and listen to Doug because he'd been around for a long time and was good at what he did. Doug had a very unique habit: anybody who was new or not as experienced as him was called Buckwheat. In all the years I knew him, he never explained why he called people Buckwheat. He just did. It was his way of letting you know your place in the pecking order.

When I met him, I said, "I'm Bob. We're going to be working together. I'm going to start working Friday nights so you'll probably see a lot of me."

"Yeah, okay. Let's go, Buckwheat." We climbed in the ambulance, one of the newer Cadillacs. Because he was senior, he got to pick out what he wanted to drive. As we climbed into the nice, new, red, white, and blue Cadillac, he looked at me and said, "We're going to be busy tonight."

Working with him and having heard the lore about his larger-than-life reputation, I was nervous but excited, because he was really well known for being what we in the business affectionately called a "shit magnet." Because he told me it was going to be busy, and because he'd already got a reputation for being a "shit magnet," I figured that night was going to be interesting. And it didn't disappoint.

We'd pulled into Dunkin' Donuts for the first of several obligatory coffee stops on a night shift when the radio crackled to life: "District 2, District 4 and any available unit identify. Shots fired Main and Albany. Multiple reports. Multiple victims and also a possible officer shot."

I reached over and grabbed the microphone. Given where we were, I knew that we were the closest of the units they had called and we were going to be the first on the scene. My voice was a little shaky. "District 2's responding. We're two minutes out. We'll advise." By the time I got that out of my face, Doug had already got the lights and the siren going. Buckwheats didn't touch those. Buckwheats could touch the radio, but Buckwheats didn't touch lights and siren switches. I was not yet worthy.

We roared down the streets, and I tried to remember the rules of triage, which is the process of prioritizing and sorting the most critical first. I'd not been in a situation with multiple victims. When you get one report, two reports, and then you add in the dynamic of, "We may have officers shot," everybody's adrenaline starts pumping.

We started watching the intersections because we knew police cruisers were going to be coming from everywhere to protect their own, so we had to make sure that we didn't get clobbered getting to the call. It was my job to look to the right out my window and clear an intersection. I'd better be right or I would probably have somebody driving through my door.

Am I going to have to choose which life to save? Am I going to have to say I don't have enough people, you're too badly injured, or you're already dead and I have to go help someone else?

All my fears and doubts chased each other through my head. Could I do this? I had just enough time to run through the questions and hang on for dear life as we careened around a maze of corners onto the scene.

There's no way you could miss it. It was a strobe light show. There were dozens of police units. Everybody wanted in on this type of call. The fire department was coming down the street from the opposite direction. And now, as we pulled onto the scene, I spotted people running toward us.

What are we doing? Who are they? Should we stop? Should we bail? Who the hell are these people and do they have guns? Is somebody going to shoot me?

Doug screeched the ambulance to a stop so we could figure out what was going on. Now we saw that one of the guys running towards us had a badge around his neck. He was in civilian clothes, but he had a badge wrapped around his neck.

Undercover cops. We're okay.

He approached Doug's side of the car and said, "Listen, we were doing a drug raid. It went bad. Take this guy first."

Two other officers ran toward us with a third guy in the middle. They also yelled, "Take this guy first."

I could see other victims in front of the ambulance, sprawled on the ground. The guy was probably not hurt that badly. Hell, he basically just ran up to us. My triage rules were telling me *this guy could wait; we'd go get the others.*

"Cops go first," Doug said. "Get in the back. Get started."

Okay. Buckwheats didn't argue. We put the detective in the back. I pulled off his army fatigue jacket and discovered he had a bullet wound in his upper bicep. It was what we call a "through and through." You can see where the bullet went. The detective's wound was a graze, not in any way life threatening.

"Did you get hit anywhere else?" I asked him.

"Nope. Just this one."

I put a sterile bandage on it and controlled the bleeding. We headed out for St. Francis, the trauma center that was down the street. The total scene time lasted a minute, minute and a half.

Not bad.

"You got any other injuries, any medical issues?" I asked the cop.

"Nope. Nothing until that asshole shot me. I got him, though. Hope the bastard's dead."

Okay.

I could hear Doug on the radio talking to the other ambulances.

"Looks like there's three others down. They're all civilians."

He no sooner got the words out of his mouth than he had to slam on the brakes to avoid hitting two more cops who were half-carrying, half-dragging a guy toward us. The Cadillac's big rear door swung open and all of a sudden a body hurtled into the ambulance. The person or body—I didn't know if he was alive or dead—landed with a thud and was now stuck in the twelve-inch space between the bench seat and the stretcher. He had missed the bench, missed the stretcher, and was now trapped between the two. My shot cop sat on the bench.

This is interesting. This is not how they taught me in class.

The cop who threw him in said, "Take him with you before the rest of the guys shoot him. He shot a cop."

My first patient was now extremely pissed off. He looked me right in the eye and said, "Don't touch him. That's the bastard that shot me."

"Look, man, I've got to work on him. You can shoot him again later if you want to, but he's in my ambulance and I have to work on him."

I was really uncomfortable now, because I was getting the glare from him while I was trying to assess my new patient. My very quick assessment revealed that the first patient, or his fellow officers, were really good shots because I could see blood coming from two holes in the patient they just threw into the truck. There were two holes in his chest, both pretty easy to find because he was bleeding through his white T-shirt.

Okay. Two bullet wounds in the chest. I can do this. What's the protocol for a guy trapped between your stretcher and your bench you can't actually get to? Oh, yeah, oxygen would be a good thing.

I looked around for an exit wound, but I couldn't really get at him to see his back. I just hoped Doug drove crazy fast, because the situation was rapidly getting ugly.

"Doug, just call ahead and tell them I need some help when I get to the ER. I'm going to need a stretcher. I can't move this guy out of here. He's stuck."

It was only going to be a couple of minutes' trip to the hospital, so I started doing a further assessment. The cop, patient number one, was breathing really quickly now because his adrenaline was running high, and he was contemplating further harm to patient number two, who was barely breathing and turning a beautiful shade of light blue, despite my stellar job with the oxygen therapy. I guessed that the bleeding in his chest cavity was claiming every bit of oxygen as fast as I could get the oxygen in.

Suddenly, the lights of the ER came into view, and for the second time in about six minutes, the back door of the ambulance was yanked open. There were frantic faces in the doorway, and I heard the security personnel and the triage nurse say, "What the hell?" They all looked at me. I didn't even get a chance to explain. They wrestled the victim out.

"He's shot twice in the chest. He's been on oxygen. He's barely breathing."

They got him onto the hospital gurney and wheeled him out into the trauma room. Doug and I grabbed the stretcher, told the cop to get on the stretcher, and followed the crowd to the opposite side of the same trauma room because that was how it happened on busy nights. Now we've got the patient who shot the cop and the cop who shot him in the same trauma room, being treated with nothing but a curtain between them. I knew the Edoc.

"What the hell happened?" the doc asked me.

I shook my head. "I can't even do it justice. You wouldn't believe me if I told you." I pointed to the cop. "He's a cop." I reached over and pointed the other way. "That guy shot him in the arm. He shot back, put two in his chest. Both of them were tossed into the ambulance by other guys with guns, and you saw where everybody landed. Now they're yours. I've got to go. My work is done."

As I turned to leave, I heard the trauma surgeon asking for the chest tray, which is never a good sign, because that means they're basically going to splay the patient's chest open in an effort to save him. I guessed the cop would have the satisfaction of seeing the outcome of his time spent at the range.

Me? I was going to clean up and get ready for whatever craziness was next, because I knew that this shooting was going to lead to more shootings before the end of the shift. It was just the way the city works. It had taken only sixteen minutes out of my life. It had seemed a whole lot longer.

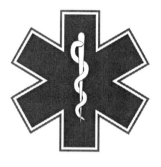

CHAPTER 4

"MY HUSBAND! MY HUSBAND!"

"MY HUSBAND! MY HUSBAND!"

I was home one night, having finally gone to bed at a normal time, when the alert pager for the fire department jarred me awake at 1:00 am for a reported structure fire in a condo. The condo was in the complex I lived in, five buildings over, so I thought I'd go directly to the scene, a department-sanctioned action. If you're closer to the scene than the firehouse, you go to the scene. I got in my car, turned the blue light on, and rolled onto the scene. I put all my turnout gear on: my helmet, fire boots, and turnout coat. *I looked good.* I ran up to the condo.

A woman stood on the front porch, pointing at the house and screaming, "My husband! My husband!"

I could see smoke and flames in the living room through the front door. "Where is he? Is he in the house? Is he hurt? Where is he?"

She was shrieking and sobbing and pointing at the house. "My husband!"

She couldn't answer. I knew I had to do a search, because I could hear on the radio that the engine hadn't signed on yet, so it was going to be a couple minutes for the guys to get to the building. The smoke was getting heavier and the flames were getting bigger, and if the guy was in there, I wouldn't have a lot of time.

I'll run in. I'll grab him. How bad can this be? These condos aren't that big. I live in one just like it, so I know the layout.

I decided to go in and start searching. This was, frankly, a very dumb move. I didn't have an air pack. I was just trying to be a hero, which was stupid. But I didn't think about that. She was screaming, and I was going to save this guy and—ta-da!—I was going to have my first kickass save.

I'll search real quickly around the base of the fire, which is in the living room near the couch and the drapes.

The drapes were starting to catch on fire and the flames were getting larger the farther in I went. I could see he was not in the chair. He was not on the floor. He was not on the couch. So, he was not in living room. He was not in the dining room, which I could barely see through the smoke.

I need to move faster.

He was not in the kitchen. He had to be upstairs. I hustled upstairs and searched from bedroom to bedroom, all over the house. The smoke was getting thicker. I started to cough. I realized my search was a dumb thing to do.

I could hear the engines coming, the sirens getting closer, and then the whoosh of air brakes outside. So, I finished the search fast. I couldn't find him. I didn't know where the hell he was. I checked the bathroom really quickly, not in the tub, not on the floor. I came down the stairs, coughing and hacking. I headed outside.

The chief pulled up and asked, "What's going on?"

I shook my head. "I did a search. She was screaming, 'My husband. My husband.' I don't know..."

Cough, cough, cough.

"I don't know where the hell he is. I can't find him."

He sent in another team with a hose line to knock down the fire, and he sent in guys with air packs to do another search for the victim. The woman was now beginning to calm down as she saw that we were putting out the fire.

The chief turned to the lady. "Ma'am, where the hell is your husband? We can't find him."

"He's in Chicago on business."

He looked at her, his eyes bulging out of his head. I whipped around so fast you could have heard my neck snap. "What?"

She said, "He's in Chicago. He's going to kill me. I'm not supposed to be smoking in the house. I fell asleep and set the couch on fire."

I really want to kill you right now.

I was coughing and hacking. The chief said, "You're going to the emergency room to get checked out for smoke inhalation."

I started to protest, but he cut me off. "It's not a discussion. It's an order. You don't need the ambulance." He assigned one of the guys to drive me over to the ER, which was only about a mile away.

After the fire he came to pick me up. As he walked into the treatment room, I started talking, fast. "It didn't look that bad when I got there. I knew the condo because it's the same as mine. I figured you guys were a couple minutes out. I'd go look—"

The chief wasn't having it. "You ever do that again, I'll kick your ass off the department. You're a risk to yourself, and you're a risk to other people because if you had gotten hurt, we would've had to send somebody in looking for you *and* for him. Do you understand me?"

"Yes, Chief."

"Good. Suck on the oxygen and then go the hell home."

That was my stupid firefighter quasi-hero move, never to be repeated. From the time a fire starts in a residential room, it takes less than five minutes to take that room from simply smoldering to fully involved, flames rolling up and over the ceiling, a temperature of 800 to 1,500 degrees, and the smoke banking down to the point where you cannot see or breathe. The smoke drops to literally less than a foot off the ground, which is why you need to cover your mouth, crawl as low as you can, and get the heck out of there.

I figured I could see how much fire there was, knew how long it was going to be before water got on it, knew how quickly I could get through the house looking for somebody, and drag his butt out the door. I figured I could beat the odds and get it done, and I didn't, because the guy I was going to rescue was…in Chicago.

Chief Persons was the quintessential small town fire chief. He was older, had lived in town for years, was real rough around the edges, a good guy, took care of his people, took care of his depart-ment, and wanted everybody to be the best, even though we weren't a very busy department. He did a good job, and he wouldn't take crap from anybody, especially not snot-nosed little old me.

At this point in my life, my schedule was a blur. Which uniform was I wearing? (I had taken yet another job, working full-time at St. Francis hospital as an EMT in the emergency room. So now I was up to four jobs, two paid and two volunteer.) Was I going to the ambulance and then to the hospital? Was I going to the hospital, then to the ambulance?

My whole life became wrapped around the work, which is pretty typical for EMTs, nurses, ER doctors, and paramedics. Our relation-ships are chunked into very short periods of time and because of this it is rare to find somebody in emergency services who has been dating or married to the same person for a long time.

It was very rare to have a day off. I'd been dating the same woman for a while. We'd go six months, then break off, go another eight months, break it off. My work was an issue. She was an outdoor person. I was so tired I wanted to be inside and just chill. We had some good chemistry in certain things, and had some not-so-great chemistry in others. She understood why I wanted to do what I was doing—she was a volunteer EMT as well—but there was the job and then there was the personal life, and we in emergency services are not generally good at prioritizing those. I know now that I wasn't. We can prioritize anything at a scene. We just can't prioritize our lives.

In many parts of this country, volunteers still provide the fire and ambulance services, although their ranks are rapidly dwindling. These folks are in the middle of a barbeque, in the middle of Christmas morning, unwrapping presents with the kids, or it's the middle of the night and they've got to go to work the next morning, but when the bell rings, they're up and out. When your neighbor's house catches fire on Christmas morning, or someone starts choking during Thanksgiving dinner, dedicated people leave their family gatherings to go help. The family whose house is burning, or whose loved one is ill is the main focus, but it's the responder's families who lose a mother, a father, or a kid, often for several hours, to handle the emergency. It disrupts the family and there are only so many times that can happen before family life starts to suffer. The more involved someone is in the service, the more time the job takes up, between training, calls, and meetings.

I know for a fact that the majority of people in any given community do not understand what EMS personnel go through so that when they dial three numbers, 9-1-1, everything falls into place. It impacts relationships, and the tentacles of the impact weave into a lot of places. It impacts work because you've fought a structure fire all night and you're going to work the next day, exhausted. You were up with a head-on collision on a winter road, and the following morning you've got to deal with a school delay and getting your kids on the bus, then getting to work, and you're trashed. The smaller the town, the more likely you are to know one of the people involved in the incident. It's a neighbor. It's a friend. It's a coworker. The teenage kid that you just pulled out of a wreck at 4:00 am is your best friend's daughter. You're emotionally and physically exhausted and when you come home, you don't want to talk. If you've never done this work, it is impossible to explain to a civilian the emotions that you go through because of what you've seen and what you've done. It takes a toll. I know that *now*.

But for me at that time, in my twenties, real life was what happened at work, and I did not recognize the toll it was taking. All I knew was that I was off Saturday night. Did I have a date or not? Was that date going to turn into Sunday morning, or was it just going to be dinner? It really didn't matter. I wasn't able to make any kind of emotional connection anyway, so it just didn't matter. I knew that there was a piece of me that was missing, but like others, I'd been trained to compartmentalize my emotions. For a long, long time, I felt as if I were almost having an out-of-body experience, watching my life rather than being connected to it. Some people drink. Some people exercise. Some people go from relationship to relationship. We all have our own coping mechanisms; those of us who don't, burn out fast.

For four years, I worked ninety-plus hours a week, either on the ambulance or in the emergency room. Many in the EMS field do the same. You've got to have a very supportive family structure or some pretty good friends that can put up with you. The problem is a lot of those good friends are in the industry, so the war stories start and you don't really get to break from it.

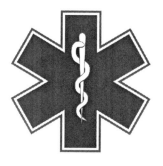

CHAPTER 5

DO YOU KNOW WHO THIS IS?

DO YOU KNOW WHO THIS IS?

I left Professional Ambulance Service and began working for L & M Ambulance, the competition in Hartford, and was still working at the ER where I met Eddie. We worked for a couple of years doing twelve-hour shifts together at the ED, then at Hunter's Ambulance, and eventually we both went to jail together (more on that in the next chapter). We also ended up becoming roommates for a while, moving to the town of Berlin and joining the Kensington Fire Department, a department that did both fire and ambulance work in town. We ended up doing more ambulance calls than anything else.

We were called out to the Berlin Turnpike for a pedestrian who had been struck, so we both hopped in my car and drove the half-mile to the firehouse, pulled in, grabbed the ambulance, and took off for the call. We arrived at the scene to find that the victim had been thrown about fifty feet from the road. He was lying at the bottom of the only tree anywhere around.

We grabbed all the gear out of the truck—backboard, collar, trauma box, oxygen—and went running over to the victim. When we got there, we saw that our victim was a uniformed police officer. Cruisers arrived, and a fire truck pulled up. We didn't know who the victim was because he was face down, but it didn't matter. When you're treating a cop, a fireman, one of your own EMTs or paramedics, or a kid, you go into overdrive. We were just about to log-roll him over when the sergeant tapped me on the shoulder and said, "It's Jeff."

My heart leaped into my throat, and I looked at Eddie. Jeff was a fellow member of the fire department, a town police officer and a former corrections officer who worked with us at the jail. He'd been on the ambulance and done calls with us. We'd even gone to the range to shoot together. He was a good friend.

We log-rolled him over and realized that he had a very significant head injury. We had a hard time getting an airway on him. His face was bloodied. His mouth was bloodied. We had to manage the airway as best we could, which involved suctioning the blood out of his airway, then putting in an artificial plastic airway to try to get an air exchange going. We get him secured to the backboard, get his head immobilized, and get him into the ambulance. We take off for the hospital, which is about a ten-minute ride away. I was in the back working on him. Eddie was driving faster than he should have been, but it was Jeff and we needed to get him there.

About five minutes into the transport, Jeff began to seize because of the head injury. I gave him oxygen. His heart was still beating, but his airway was filling with blood. I had the Ambubag, a large plastic cylinder about the size of a football that fills with oxygen and has a clear mask that goes over the patient's face. You put the mask over the patient's face, hold it as securely as you can, and then squeeze the bag to force air into the patient's lungs. The problem was that I only had a small plastic airway holding his airway open, and blood still had to be suctioned out from around it, and now he was seizing! I got into a rhythm, squeezed the bag five times to get in as much oxygen as possible, took it off, suctioned the blood out to make room, and put it back on. Five times, back and forth, back and forth.

Eddie...drive faster.

Jeff had some fractures, but I wasn't even going to spend time splinting them at that point because he was seizing, and I had nothing to give him to make the seizures stop. I knew that the seizures were indicative of a really severe head injury. We had a police escort in front of the ambulance, and we had a police escort behind the ambulance, blocking traffic, trying to get us to the hospital as quickly as possible. Ed had the pedal to the floorboard, and we burned through the city of Meriden.

We got to the hospital, and Jeff was still seizing. Eddie, me, and everyone around us had tears running down our faces. We knew.

Jeff made it into the evening and then passed away from the head injury. He was the first police officer killed in the line of duty in the town of Berlin's history.

Afterward, Eddie and I just sat in the back of the ambulance. It was so frustrating to not be able to do anything. We didn't have the skill set or the tools to save him, not the drugs or the IVs. There was nothing more that we, as EMTs, could do. At that point, I committed to advancing my skills; I knew I had to be better than that.

We found out the rest of the story later: Jeff had pulled over to help a disabled vehicle and was setting out flares when a drunk driver struck him and sent him flying. Then the driver drove into the guardrail. He was so out of it he had no idea what he had done. From that point forward, I have had absolutely no sympathy for drunk drivers. None. The drunks walk away, but they wreak havoc in their wake and don't even know what they've done. If I'm driving down the road and I think somebody is under the influence, I'll follow that car. I'll call 9-1-1 and stay on the line and talk the cops into that car's location.

Later on in my career I responded to a motor vehicle accident in which a drunk had plowed into a vehicle and killed a father and a young daughter. The drunk was unbelievably belligerent, screaming, "I know my rights!" and just being an all-around pain in the ass. The people he hit were annihilated; there was absolutely nothing we could do for them. The drunk walked away from the crash unscathed. The state trooper, a good friend, had him cuffed, but this guy was spitting on the trooper and giving him grief. I snapped. I grabbed the drunk by the arm, and I walked him away from the cruiser. All I heard in the background was, "Don't hurt him. He's in custody."

I walked him over to the car he had hit, grabbed him by the scruff of the neck, shoved his head through the window where he could see the two bodies in the car: "This is what you did, you stupid asshole." I made him look. He sobered up really quickly, and threw up all over the place. I handed him back to the trooper. "I'm done." The trooper just stood there shaking his head at me.

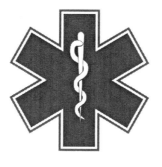

CHAPTER 6

OFF TO JAIL

OFF TO JAIL

After about eleven months at Hunter's, Eddie decided that he wanted to work for the Connecticut Department of Corrections. I followed suit because the Department of Corrections was looking for medical personnel to work in the jails, and they were paying three times more money than we were making working two jobs on the ambulance. So, I left the ambulance business full-time for a few years and did my medicine and my emergency responses working in a maximum-security jail, working an eight to sixteen-hour shift five days a week.

I learned very quickly how to deal with overdoses, people who were detoxing, and patients who were all manner of crazy. I went to the Corrections Academy for eight weeks of training, where we learned hand-to-hand combat. We learned the laws. We learned correctional techniques such as handcuffing, fingerprinting, and search techniques—not only the body searches we had to do on each inmate at intake, but also how to search cell blocks for weapons.

When working in the jail, I would carry a radio and nothing else. I found out quickly I had to be hyper aware and use wits, not weapons. We didn't carry handcuffs, a nightstick, or a Taser, because they could all be taken and used against us. I learned quickly how to communicate and project authority, tough for a twenty-three-year-old kid, but everything you did in dealing with those guys was about respect and talking your way through situations. Otherwise, you had to be prepared to defend yourself at a moment's notice.

It's a spooky feeling, the very first time you walk through that heavy steel door and it clangs shut behind you. You realize that you're locked in and somebody has to let you out too. I used to say, "I'm doing time eight hours at a whack."

The culmination of that training was to be treated like an inmate for twenty-four hours. We were brought in in handcuffs. They went through a whole intake procedure: we were strip-searched, put into prison-issue clothes, and then locked up in this old jail facility for twenty-four hours, two people to a cell. They had corrections officers who played the roles of warden and corrections officers. We had to go to meals. They would search us as we were coming out of the mess hall to make sure we hadn't stolen forks, knives, or spoons, anything that could be turned into homemade weapons. The door to our jail cell and the cell next to ours did not operate properly. It was an unused facility so it was in disrepair, but it was good enough for training purposes. The guy who played the warden for our class was going out of his way to be obnoxious. My cellmate for the evening, Ricky, and I worked it out with the two guys in the other cell so that when the "warden" came by, we'd take him hostage. They wanted to treat us like inmates; we'd act like inmates. When the guy came by later that evening and began giving us grief, we slid the door open and grabbed him.

The corrections officers who were managing the class didn't know what to do, because there wasn't a SWAT team to call in.

"All right. Come on, guys. You've got to knock it off."

We held him for three hours and wouldn't let him go. It had never happened before. Ricky actually went on to become a warden.

After graduation, I was assigned to the Morgan Street Jail, a repository for folks who had already been arraigned in court and held over for trial, as well as people who had been newly arrested by the Hartford Police Department. The PD would roll in with handcuffed suspects and then transfer custody to us. Those folks had been picked up off the street only minutes before, so they could be drunk, under the influence of drugs, crazy, or violent. The charges against those folks ranged from drunk and disorderly to "this guy just committed a double murder."

We would process each one—search, fingerprint, breathalyze—wrestle with the uncooperative ones, and then put them all in a big 40 x 40 holding cell until we had a smaller cell for them.

Some of them would have to stay with us over a weekend, depending on when they had been arrested. Others would be able to make bail fairly quickly and leave. The folks coming in on Friday night stayed for the weekend, because they couldn't go to court to see a judge until Monday. As they would come down from being drunk or high, going through drug or alcohol withdrawal, they would have lots of hallucinations.

I remember one particular guy who was wedged in the corner of a cell. These were the old-style jail cells, 8 x 10 feet, three concrete-block walls, and a door with steel bars. This guy was screaming, "Kill them! Kill them! Kill them!"

I'll play.

"Kill what?"

"Kill the spiders. Kill the spiders," and he smacked himself, smacked the bed, smacked the wall, and he bounced from side to side, and curled up in a ball in the corner of the cell. *He* could see spiders; these spiders were real to him. "It's right there. Get that one. Get that one!"

I now smacked jail cell bars, trying to get this guy to calm down. "Did I get him?"

"No. He's over there."

"Okay. I'll get him."

I finally got a couple of other correction officers to come over, and we opened the door. As we entered, he came charging at us because he wanted out of where all these spiders were. Now we had to restrain him and wrestle him while he screamed, "They're on me! They're on me! They're on me!" He banged his head on the concrete wall while we tried to cuff him. He shrieked, "They're going to eat me!"

I'm concerned at this point he was going to end up with a head injury.

Lots of paperwork—bad.

We finally got him down, and the officers sat on him while I went to the medication cabinet to grab a syringe of Haldol, or vitamin H as it's known. I injected it into his arm, and he finally calmed down. We had to medicate him for the next forty-eight hours to get him through the withdrawal period so he didn't have another psychotic episode.

That was one challenge of working in the jail.

The other challenge of working in the jail was that I used to work noon to 8 pm, so guys who came in and made bail would get back out into the community. When I got off at eight at night, I would go to work from either nine or ten at night until seven the next morning on the ambulance. It was not at all uncommon for me to have deal with a guy in the jail during my noon to eight shift and come across him and his buddies on the street several hours later when I was on an ambulance call. I'd walk onto the scene and hear "Hey CO." I'd turn around and have a moment of fear. Was this

"Hey, CO, I'm going to kick your ass"? More often than not, it was, "Hey, CO, I remember you."

My philosophy was that I could make a mistake the next day and land in jail just as easily as some of those guys, so I treated everyone with the level of respect they gave me. Most people don't realize that it's not necessarily always habitual criminals who end up in prison or in jail. Any one of us could do something accidentally, have a lapse of judgment, and end up there. By treating everybody with as much respect as they gave me, I didn't have too many issues.

I spent about ten months at Morgan Street, and then moved over to what they affectionately called the Community Correctional Center, which was a much larger jail in Hartford, and I worked there for another three and a half years. I transferred from being a medic to being a full corrections officer, mostly because I wanted the overtime. When I got over there, the inmate population in that facility was five hundred, and I became a block officer. I was also often assigned to the emergency response team within the facility for my shift.

The blocks, or housing units, in the jail were set up like a plus sign, with a control room the size of a toll collector's booth in the middle, and four tiers, as they were called. Each tier held fifteen inmates in twelve cells and had a day room where inmates ate all three meals, could play cards, or watch the TV. There were sliding glass doors that would slide slowly open or closed and clang into place to block off each of the tiers. As the block officer, I would have to separate each of the areas by opening or closing doors to allow inmates in or out of their cells, their tiers, or the block itself.

The rules were you could never have more than two inmates out on a tier at a time, and the rest of the doors were supposed to be shut so that the inmates were contained. The only exception was at meal times, when you would open all the cell doors, and everyone had to go into the dayroom to be fed.

Also, once an hour on every shift, you had to do what was called tripping the block. You had to make a trip around, so you'd have to go into the unit control booth and close all the doors except for the door to the tier you were going to walk down. None of the inmates could be out at that point; they all had to be secured in their cells or they had to be secured in the day room. You had to walk down and physically look in every cell and make sure that everybody was accounted for and okay, because you never knew when somebody would try to commit suicide or an inmate would get sick. It had to be done once an hour and that took a while because you had to go down, do one tier, come back, close that door, open another door, and then trip that piece of the block. It would take fifteen minutes once an hour.

Working on the emergency response team, I'd respond to fights, or medical emergencies. I spent a lot of time on the response team because it made sense to have a medically trained officer available, especially since most of the others just had basic CPR or first aid and I was an EMT. I worked the midnight shift and nearly every morning I'd be running to deal with fights. The guys could be fighting because one guy got three pancakes and the other guy got two. You fight for everything in prison: pancakes, TV choices, and your life.

Sometimes the intersection between my two careers made for interesting times. The first day I showed up as a medic, I was told it was an all-male facility. I had to do medication rounds.

Because inmates are wards of the state, they continue to take whatever medications they were taking when they got arrested. I had a file with cards listing the inmate's name and number and the medications that had been preportioned into cups. The inmate would come to the window, and I'd confirm that he was the right inmate and watch him take the medication.

A few minutes into med call, this person came sashaying down the walkway, his T-shirt tied up above the midriff. He had a slender build, very, very tight pants, painted toenails, painted fingernails, and very small breasts.

They said it was an all-male facility. Hmm.

"Hello. You must be the new one," she (?) said.

"Your name?"

"My name's Gloria."

"I don't have medication for Gloria."

Everybody started cracking up.

Okay. This is play a trick on the new guy. I got it.

I turned to the medic who was orienting me, and he said, "George."

"George who?"

I found the card and I looked at the medication: hormones. George was in the process of going through sex change therapy when he was arrested and the State of Connecticut correctional system was continuing the therapy under court order.

"Gloria" was released a few days later.

Later in the week, my partner and I were on ambulance duty in the city, cruising through an area where a fair amount of hooker traffic worked the streets. As we drove down the street, my partner looked over and said, "Whoa. She's *actually* good looking. She's new."

"Really? She's a hooker. Leave it. Stop. Don't even look over there."

They would always harass us. We'd drive by and they'd call out, "Hey, you guys want a date? You've got a bed in the back."

We'd slowed down, approaching the corner, and he was still talking about this girl, so I looked over. She wore a very short skirt and very high heels. She had a fairly trim figure, hair done up, nails done up. As we pulled up to the stop sign about to take the turn around the corner where she stood, I got a good look at the face, and I realized who it was: Gloria/George. At this point I stopped the truck, and said to my partner, "Do you want to go talk to her?"

He said, "No. I was just admiring the view from the back."

"Do you want me to tell you a secret? That's a guy."

"No, it's not."

"Yes, it is. I can't tell you how I know, but if you get under that nice miniskirt, there is a nasty surprise."

He just kind of looked at me. "The jail, right?"

I shrugged. "All I can say is she's not what you think she is."

We left.

In the four and a half years I worked there, I ended up being investigated twice by Internal Affairs for excessive force charges. In one case, we needed to restrain this guy who didn't want to be locked up, didn't want to take a shower, didn't want to do anything. We ended up sending the response team in, and he was so strong it took all eight of us to hold him. He claimed that people were choking him. I was the one at his head, so I went to the Internal Affairs investigation, and the investigating officer said, "It's alleged that you choked this inmate."

"Well, number one, if I had choked him, it wouldn't have taken eight guys to fight him because he'd be unconscious. Number two, the guy was lying on his stomach while we were trying to cuff his hands behind his back, and I was holding his head to prevent him from biting anybody, but I held his head in a position that kept his airway open. I wasn't choking him."

"What do you mean?"

There was a CPR poster on the wall behind his head.

I said, "Turn around. Look at the diagram of the choking victim."

"Yeah?"

"Now picture that diagram of the person as if he were on his stomach. What position was his head in?"

"Oh."

"Are we done?"

"Yes. We're done."

"Okay."

The second incident involved a block officer who had left one too many doors open, including the dayroom door. He opened the corridor door to trip the block with eight inmates in the dayroom. He was grabbed, pulled into the dayroom and pinned in the corner. He was able to hit a panic alarm and everybody came running because a panic alarm means an officer is in trouble.

Another officer and I responded first. The inmates had broken the TV antenna off of the television and one guy had it in his hand. He wasn't pointing it at the officer, but there was enough of a threat in our minds. The two of us came in at a dead run, yelling at him to "Drop the weapon," which he didn't do, so we both hit the guy at the same time like a football tackle, sending him crashing into the wall. He ended up needing almost a hundred stitches and had a concussion.

Into Internal Affairs again we went. The investigating officer was different but had the same attitude. "The inmate was injured. Can you explain why you used excessive force?"

Clearly, we'd moved from being under investigation to being guilty without an interim stop at "What happened?"

I said, "Quite frankly, I'd have been within my rights to have killed the inmate. He was holding an officer hostage, brandishing a weapon in a correctional facility, and he failed to drop the weapon after we yelled three times for him to drop it as we were running in. We had a hostage situation; he was in the commission of multiple felonies within a correctional facility, endangering the life and safety of an officer. We could have killed him and been justified. All we did was knock him down."

"Well, um."

"No. Let's list out the felonies that he was committing. I've got four. He's got four additional charges that we can bring against him, and you're here taking up my time because he's got some stitches and a concussion? The officer's fine and everybody else just sat down and didn't want to play after we took the situation under control."

"Well, what did you say when you ran in the room?"

"'Drop the weapon. Drop the weapon. Drop the weapon.' Then we dropped him. Are we done?"

"Well, we're done for now."

"Good, because I'm done talking about it. I've got to go finish the paperwork, because I'm still figuring out how many new charges we're going to hit this guy with. We're adding at least the four felony charges. The state police will be here to rearrest him tomorrow. You guys do what you want, but we're not dropping the issue and we don't see it as an issue."

I was in and out of a long-term relationship at this point, the "out" parts being because I was not really a nice person during those four years. I was very paranoid. When inmates told me, "We'll see you on the outside," I'd say, "Yeah, yeah, whatever." I just chalked it up to posturing in front of the other inmates.

There was a time when I took a couple of days off and moved from Berlin, Connecticut, to Meriden, Connecticut. I came back into the jail on my next day on. I had been working the same block for probably about three weeks, so I'd gotten to know most of the inmates there. I had not even gone into the office to see my sergeant to give him my new phone number and address, all the stuff you're mandated to tell the department. I'd been on the block for about fifteen minutes when one of the guys came up to me and said, "How do you like Meriden?"

I asked him, "What do you mean?"

"Well you live in Meriden now, don't you?"

It struck me at that point that not only could the "We'll see you on the outside" be real, but there was a network that I had not appreciated: the guys inside were connected outside the walls of the jail as efficiently as they had been when they had been on the outside. I obtained a pistol permit. For the remainder of my time with the corrections department, I was not without a firearm at arm's reach twenty-four hours a day. I went to work armed. I went home armed. Everywhere I went I carried a weapon. On the ambulance, I wasn't able to carry a firearm, but I did carry other forms of self-defense, just in case.

I was paranoid and pissed at the world because I was working so many hours a week, and I was not in a good place to be in a relationship with anybody. That fact manifested itself at one point when I was sleeping, and the girl I was living with came up behind me to wake me up. As she put her hand on my back and neck, in my half-asleep state, I actually picked her up and threw her across the room. I'd immediately snapped into self-defense mode, believing somebody was grabbing me. It became glaringly clear to both of us at that moment that I was not a good person to be in a relationship with. I didn't realize just how squirrely I was getting until that happened. I would blow through my sick time. I would blow through my vacation time as fast as I'd get it, because I was working sixty-four hours a week at the jail, and another twenty-four on the ambulance. But when that incident with my girlfriend happened, it was a wake-up call.

Very shortly thereafter, I was injured on the job and out for about thirty-five weeks. I had torn a ligament in my wrist on a malfunctioning cell lock. They didn't have anything that qualified as light duty at the jail, so I couldn't go back to work until I was declared 100 percent functional. During my recuperation, I was notified that I'd been accepted into a paramedic training program, so I attended the first fifteen weeks with a cast on my wrist.

When I went back to the jail, I went to my lieutenant and said, "I'm resigning, effective immediately."

I could have easily stayed with the Department of Corrections, done twenty-five years, and had a great retirement. But after being away from the jail for thirty-five weeks, I realized how paranoid I'd become, and how much different and better my life was when I was away from there.

A lot of fortuitous things have happened throughout my career that have really been guideposts. I spent a total of four and a half years with the Corrections Department. I learned a lot about how to deal with people, such as how to quickly defuse potentially explosive situations by using my head and my mouth, rather than fists and writing people up. I learned how to be a good communicator to get myself out of trouble quickly. I learned a different kind of medicine by dealing with lots of withdrawals and medication-related issues. However, those are four and a half years I'd never want to repeat.

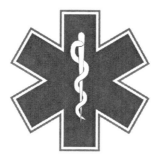

CHAPTER 7

CELLITIS

CELLITIS

My jail career provided me with its own kind of education. Things in corrections have changed dramatically, but back in the 1980s, psychologically troubled inmates were mixed in with general population until they began to act up, at which point they would be removed to specialized areas of the jail such as the medical ward. If they were really problematic to the point that they were trying to injure themselves or set fire to a cell, they would sometimes be put on suicide watch or put in a strip cell.

Suicide watch means that somebody had to physically look at them every fifteen minutes throughout the day and log that they were okay. If they were in a strip cell, they were checked every thirty minutes. A strip cell is an 8x8 cell, with a metal door and a peephole with a plastic window. The inmates were either naked or dressed only in underwear, because anything they were given could be used as a weapon. The room contained a metal bed that was bolted to the floor and had a paper-thin mattress, and there was a stainless steel metal toilet/sink combination that was also bolted down. That didn't stop inmates from ripping the sink/toilet unit off the wall and flooding the cells. Typically, they were given a single roll of one-ply, government-issue toilet paper. Occasionally, they'd rip the mattress apart, so we'd take that out of the cell too.

I did the intake on a new inmate deemed as a danger to himself but not to others. He wasn't considered suicidal, so he was put in a strip cell. We had checked him several times during my shift. Then it was time for me to leave. I was gone for sixteen hours. I came back the next day and the cell was empty.

"Where'd he go?"

"He's in the hospital. He tried to kill himself and he damned near made it."

"With what? There was nothing in the cell."

The officer I was relieving said, "You wouldn't believe me if I told you. You know the roll of toilet paper, right? He used that."

The inmate had taken six-foot lengths of toilet paper, pulled them off and lined them up on the floor. The officers looking in just ignored it: What can anybody do with single-ply toilet paper? He was being quiet, not annoying anybody. Somebody noticed that he was taking the ends of the toilet paper and rolling them into a very fine strip. No big deal there, they figured. Let him have his fun.

What nobody saw was that he was doing this with the entire roll of toilet paper. He had about fifteen or twenty of these six-foot, now very tightly wound pieces of paper of straw wrapper like consistency. When you braid those together, do you know how strong it gets? Neither did we. He braided them together and made a rope. He then ran the rope around the ventilation duct in the cell ceiling and tried to strangle himself in the period between officers' visits.

Everybody had done what they were supposed to do. This guy was smart enough to know the rules, but also crazy enough to do this. He ended up almost killing himself with one-ply toilet paper. I didn't believe it was possible until we had the evidence bag with the "rope" in it, and we were able to pull on his toilet-paper rope. It held together.

I've seen more than a few suicides in my career. The youngest suicide I dealt with was fourteen. I've come across all kinds of suicide methods: pills, gas, guns, hanging. One kid committed suicide by pouring gas inside his car and then driving ninety miles an hour into a bridge abutment where he blew the car up.

The one thing that people always feel bad about when there's a suicide is, "I wish I could have done something. What were the signs? Why didn't I see it? Why didn't he tell me or she tell me?"

We often miss the signs that someone is contemplating suicide, but a lot of people just don't want to be on the planet anymore. You'll never see a sign. You'll never know. When they want to leave, they're going to leave, and there's nothing you can do to stop it. No amount of talking is going to do it.

Another thing I learned about along the way is a very strange phenomenon that occurs, especially on weekends, in jails and police lockups all around the country: prisoners like to fake seizures as a way of getting out of jail. On a Friday or Saturday night, the ER is a much nicer place to be than sitting in an 8x10 cell with a potentially stinky roommate. I have affectionately dubbed this phenomenon "cellitis."

While we can't assume that someone is faking, there are some very specific things that happen when most people have seizures. For instance, most people have either localized tremors in parts of their body, or they have full body tremors. Typically when a person is having a full-blown or grand mal seizure they're also incontinent, meaning they pee their pants. The really good fakers, will have the full body tremors, they'll flop around on the floor like a fish out of water, and they will knowingly pee to enhance the illusion that they're having a problem. It's up to us to determine who's faking.

One particular guy, Dennis, who tried it, was someone I knew well from encounters in jail and on the street. I knew, number one, he had no history of seizures. I also knew that he had been arrested on Friday night, so he was going to be incarcerated for the whole weekend, go to court on Monday morning, and might or might not be remanded back to jail by the court, which was more than likely because he didn't have a place of residence or a shot at getting someone to post his bail.

I reported to the police lockup and found him in his cell, flopping around on the floor and looking like a very sick person.

"Dennis, what's going on?"

He'd flop around some more and then he'd stop. I'd talk to him and then he'd flop around some more. He reminded me of one of those battery-operated fish that flap their fins when you make a noise. When I wasn't talking to him, he'd stop, and when I'd started to talk to him, he'd flop again. He had an audience now: three cops, the two guys from the fire department ambulance service, and me.

His eyes were closed, because all seizure patients have closed eyes.

"Watch this." I held up my fingers and waved my arms as if I were conducting a symphony. Then I stopped talking and Dennis stopped flopping. I held my fingers up again and repeated the process. At this point, everybody knew he was faking, and everybody giggled because this was now no longer a serious medical issue. This was just stupidity, cellitis.

I said to one of the officers, "Do me a favor. Grab me one of the big needles in my kit, that one right there. That's the eyeball needle. Give me that one."

All of a sudden the flopping stopped again, because Dennis really wanted to listen to what was going to happen. I start rustling the package to make it sound as if I were opening it. "I need one of you guys to come over here and pull his eyelids open because I really need a clean shot at this. When I stick this needle into his eyeball, we can see what color the fluid is and then we'll know what kind of seizure he's having."

Miraculously Dennis opened his eyes and said, "I'm good. I'm good."

"Dennis, you're feeling better?"

"Yeah, man. I'm good. I'm feeling a whole lot better now."

That became my trademark treatment when I was 100 percent sure someone was faking. Nothing works like breaking out the old eyeball needle to bring a guy around. And no, there really is no such thing as an eyeball needle. But don't tell anyone.

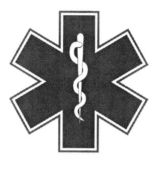

CHAPTER 8

TWO SISTERS

TWO SISTERS

I was four, maybe five years into my career when I responded to a call that was a game changer. I wasn't ready for this call. I'd seen a lot of patients by the time I received this call, but none of them were as severely hurt as this one, which came out of the blue. In fact, I wasn't even supposed to be working that day; I was covering as a favor for someone else.

It was a beautiful, sunny day; nothing going on—no storms, no wet roads, nothing. The radio barked, "Unit 453, respond priority one to the area of Farmington and Prospect for a motor vehicle accident with serious injuries. Multiple reports." Any time you hear the words "multiple reports," you know you're going to be working. A call with multiple reports means lots of people saw the accident. It also means you're going to have a lot of bystanders. The intersection of Farmington and Prospect is the dividing line between the City of Hartford and the Town of West Hartford. One side of Prospect Avenue is Hartford; the other side of Prospect is West Hartford. I didn't know which side we were going to. I didn't know which fire department we were going to be responding with.

As we came up Farmington Avenue, I could see cruisers, and West Hartford's ladder truck pulling in. It had the Jaws of Life on it. The scene was actually a block past the reported intersection and definitely in West Hartford. As we pulled in, I saw this little aqua-colored Datsun station wagon wedged up against the telephone pole, with a brown car stuck in the passenger door. I could tell that the brown car had hit the little station wagon and the momentum had pushed the station wagon into the telephone pole. One of the firemen came over to us as we grabbed our gear.

The guys in West Hartford are great, a very experienced department.

The guy who came over to meet us was pale, and firemen don't get pale.

This is not going to be good.

He said, "You're just not going to believe this. I can't believe the damage on this car, and we know for a fact this was a low-speed crash. One of our cops witnessed it. There are two people trapped in the car."

"Can we get at them?"

"Not yet. We've got to get the brown car out of the way because you can't get in the passenger side. It's too devastated. We've got to winch the car away from the telephone pole with the fire truck."

They worked quickly, and as they did so, I looked through the windshield and I honestly couldn't believe what I was seeing. The passenger side of the car was caved in about three feet so that the passenger door was pushed all the way to the center console of the car. There was a passenger in the front seat. She had been pushed over, and I could see two bodies and two heads, one underneath the other. The driver's door was up against the telephone pole. The passenger door and all of that side of the car wedged them in so they were encased in this car.

As soon as they were able to get the car back a couple of feet, they put blocks under the wheels to prevent it from rolling. They popped the driver's door with the Jaws of Life and said, "Okay. Go ahead. They're all yours."

In the opening where the driver's door once was I saw two girls, both in their twenties. The torso of one girl was wedged in by the steering wheel. The torso of the other girl, the passenger, was underneath the first and their legs were intertwined like a human pretzel, one on top of the other. The steering wheel had crumpled on them a little bit so we couldn't move them. The fireman said, "We're going to cut the windshield off. Then we're going to wrap chains around the steering column and we're going to pull it up."

Standard procedure; I know that from being a firefighter.

He continued, "We're going to cover them over with a blanket. What are you going to do?"

"I'm going to start treating them."

I reached over and started assessing the patients. The girl underneath didn't have a pulse. The girl on top was semiconscious and moaning, and I tried to figure out what she was saying. I soon realized she was calling the other girl's name. "We're taking care of both of you," I told her, and she mumbled. I gave her some oxygen and she woke up a little bit more and told me that the other girl was her sister. The one who was seriously injured but still alive was on top, her sister underneath her. I knew that there was nothing we could do for this other girl because I could see the injuries. She had been catastrophically damaged in the crash. She had an open chest wound. She had an open head wound, and I could see brain matter and blood on the door. She fit every criterion for presumption of death on the scene. But we couldn't get either one of them out until the firemen had finished unwrapping the car from around them.

I looked at the cop standing there, and I gave him a thumbs-down sign and pointed to my watch so he would note the time I had presumed her dead.

Now we had to figure out how to get the other sister out without getting her too upset, because I couldn't tell her that her sister was dead. As the firefighters pulled the dashboard away to give me more room to work, I realized that we had to untangle her legs, which were broken. I knew it would hurt and I had to tell her it was going to hurt. We also have to get a backboard under her, but we couldn't disturb the body of the other girl because we needed to preserve that as much as possible for the autopsy, photos, and crash investigation.

It took us about twenty-five minutes to get all this done, and the girl was still crying for her sister. She gained a little more consciousness because we'd given her oxygen. I was able to get an IV in. We were intermediate technicians at that time, so the only thing I could do for her was put fluid in her; I didn't have any pain management drugs. I was not yet a paramedic. Nobody in Hartford was.

We finally got her out. Another ambulance came to take charge of the other sister once we left. A crowd stood around, probably fifty people watching all of this, and I hoped that nobody said anything like, "They just presumed her," or "She's dead," or anything like that about the sister, because I was trying to keep my patient calm. Every time she'd call her sister's name, I'd say, "We're doing everything we can for her. Let's focus on you. Where else do you hurt? Squeeze my hand if you can hear me."

As I worked through all this chaos, this idiot came up and said, "I'm a doctor. Can I help?"

I say, "idiot," because broken plastic, and pieces of metal and windshield glass lay everywhere, and he was standing on this glass, next to me, *in bare feet*. The accident had happened in front of his house and he had run out to help. I didn't even know what to say to him at that point.

"One, you can leave me alone. Two, you can go put some shoes on, because I don't need another patient right now. When you're done with putting your shoes on, don't come back. That would be a big help."

"I don't think you understood. I said I'm a doctor."

"I don't care, unless you're a trauma surgeon. Are you?"

"No."

I looked at the cop and motioned for him to move the doctor back. A sea of glass and he was out there in bare feet. Idiot!

Under the circumstances help would have been great, but not when that help is getting in the way and making matters worse.

We finally got the girl out of the car, on the backboard, and into the ambulance, and we took off for St. Francis, which was probably three miles down the road. She survived. She had a broken lower leg, a broken pelvis, multiple rib fractures, and a collapsed lung.

At the end of that call, there was so much adrenaline coursing through me as I cleaned up the truck, put it back together again, and restocked the trauma bag that my hands were shaking. I sat back for a second, reliving all of what we had just gone through in the last thirty-five minutes on a bright, sunny day.

The story was they were going to work. One was driving the other to work and they were in a hurry, so the driver took a left against the light, and this other car started up from a dead stop at the traffic light, went about a hundred feet, and hit them. Their car was a newer model, mostly sheet metal; the other car, an older model, was solid steel. The cop estimated it to be about a thirty-mile-an-hour crash, but it did devastating damage. None of us had ever seen damage like that in a car that was not involved in a high-speed crash.

Thinking about it afterward, I realized that if I could manage that level of devastation and complexity and deal with the idiot with the bare feet and a crowd of watching bystanders, I could do this job. I thought about the amazing level of skill and professionalism I'd seen during the call; how the fire department, the police, everybody came together. I knew that this was a group that I wanted to be affiliated with for a long time. What was very frustrating to me at that point, personally and professionally, was the limit of our patient treatment options. We needed to finish medic training and get on the streets.

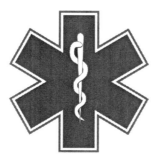

CHAPTER 9

WILLIE

CHAPTER NINE

WILLIE

As good as I was feeling about what I was doing, I realized I was working way too much. I'd always loved going to Vermont, so I bought myself a timeshare up in Stowe. For the next couple of years I took time off around my birthday to unplug. I only managed to get a full week once.

My personal life was still stuck at next to nil. I'd been seeing the same woman for nearly six years, and we'd finally realized we were completely different people and had agreed to move on. I ended up moving out, getting an apartment, and starting over.

Professionally, the severity of the calls we were getting—shootings, stabbings—was escalating. Collectively everyone involved in EMS in Hartford realized that we needed to step up our level of patient care. The emergency room directors of Hartford's three hospitals got together and agreed to offer a paramedic training course, which they cooperatively put together. About fifty people applied from within the ranks of the greater Hartford EMS community. Twenty-four of us originally started the program. We began what was a eight-month course of study, all of us still working full-time and rearranging schedules so we could get to the classes.

At the same time, Hartford Hospital decided that it wanted to go into the air ambulance business. They were training the first group of flight nurses for the Lifestar program. Quite often our classes would come together, so the first group of flight nurses and the first group of paramedics trained together. The best thing about the program was that, because it was a first time, cooperative program, the heads of departments came into lecture. The heads of the neurology, respiratory, anesthesiology, obstetrics, emergency medicine, and psychology departments all came in to teach us. The chief trauma surgeons from each hospital were actively involved. We had the best Hartford had to offer and a phenomenal educational experience. From my perspective, the education was like starting from the ground up. The level of anatomy and physiology we were expected to learn was very complex, literally thousands of pages. I'd look at the other people from my company who'd entered the program with me and wonder just how big a bite we'd taken, working full time and going to school four days a week. When it began, I was still working with the remnants of my injury from the Corrections Department, so I took notes with an injured wrist. I couldn't work road shifts either, so I began dispatching at night. I tried to give my classmates a break, putting them on the last truck out so they could study, sleep, or whatever they needed to do. We all worked all night and had to be back to class at nine in the morning.

For the first five months, we took practical lab courses, practicing intubation (putting breathing tubes into a patient's throat), working on the mannequin until we could do it in fifteen seconds or less. We had to be able to start IVs. We had to be able to do medication calculations, know which medications were appropriate and which ones were contraindicated because they'd cause the patient harm.

After the first five months of classroom training and skills sessions four or five days a week, we went into the hospitals to spend time in the emergency room, in the operating room, in the OB/

GYN suite, the psychiatric suite, and the intensive care unit. We were evaluated every step of the way by the clinical coordinators to make sure we were not only learning the stuff, but that we could actually apply it. That's when we started to lose a few people. We started with twenty-four; twenty graduated.

After the clinical training in the hospital, we had to take our knowledge to the streets. We had to use our skills under the watchful eyes of senior paramedics. On every call we had to tell them what we wanted to do, and why we wanted to do it. They would quiz us mercilessly:

"If it's this heart rhythm on the monitor, but the patient looks like this and they're taking these medications, what can't you give them?"

"Hang on."

"Don't give me 'hang on.' You're in the back of the ambulance. You've only got thirty seconds to figure this out."

I was assigned to one paramedic preceptor who walked in on the very first day and said, "I've been a paramedic for seven years and you don't know anything, but you will when you leave." I had been in EMS at this point for about the same amount of time but wasn't about to say so.

"Yes, sir. I understand."

He then went to the paramedic unit that we were going to ride with for the day, pulled out the spare drug box, opened it up, turned it upside down, and dumped absolutely everything out on the floor. Boxes with prefilled syringes, IV tubing, IV solutions, bandages, IV catheters and thirty-seven different medications in different vials and ampules were now on the floor in a big pile of glass and plastic. He took the now-empty drug box, handed it to me, and said, "Start putting that back together again. I'm going to go get a cup of coffee."

As I reassembled the drug box, he would come in and sit with his arms crossed, his cup of coffee on the table, feet up, rocking back and forth in the conference room chair. "What have you got in your hand?"

I'd read it to him.

He'd say, "Tell me what it's used for; tell me what its contraindications are; and tell me how it's administered."

I did. If I were right, he'd say, "Move on." If I were wrong, he'd say, "Go get your book and study it."

He did this to me twice in my week with him. I learned everything in that box upside down, inside out. I knew it by sight; I knew it by shape, so that when I was working in the ambulance and I had a partner who might not have been as experienced, I could say, "Hand me the Lidocaine. It's in the third compartment in the top tray." In hindsight it was great training, and as I became a paramedic preceptor later on in my career, I had to thank him for that knowledge, even though, as I lived through it, my future gratitude wasn't first on my mind.

I didn't dump the boxes out on my students, but I did make them go through the drug box every single shift. I made sure that they went through and checked the expiration dates on the medications. I would make them pull something out of a particular tray. "Tell me the indications, the contraindications. What can't you use?"

Once we were done with that five months of education, about two months of clinical rotations through all of the different departments of the hospital, and then another month or so riding on the medic units with preceptors, we were deemed worthy to graduate and take to the streets as medics in the City of Hartford.

John, one of the guys I went to paramedic school with, took a night shift with me. We weren't too far into the shift when the police dispatcher announced, "Unit 463, respond priority one. A possible shooting." It was in a notorious housing project, long since torn down, but then a hotbed of drugs, gang wars, and murder.

It was raining, and the reflections of the red and white lights danced off the buildings as we raced down the wet streets. Sirens screamed a warning to the very few people who dared to walk the street at night. We made a final turn and the scene came into view. There was a lone police car, its light bar extinguished so as not to call attention to itself. We followed suit and shut our lights and siren off as we approached. In the center of the rain-soaked street, a crowd had gathered. A woman was screaming, held up by friends or family. A man lay crumpled in the middle of the road next to his wheelchair. The cop looked nervous as we rolled to a stop and stepped out of the ambulance. "He's been shot—a lot," he shouted from about ten feet away.

The decibel level immediately increased from the crowd of distraught onlookers. We knew we would have to work quickly to save the patient and get away from the scene for our own safety. We grabbed the heart monitor, oxygen, trauma bag, and stretcher for the fourth time on this shift, and once again we waded into chaos.

I remember being surprised that there was only one cop on the scene, because this typically was a show-of-force area. The problem with this kind of situation is the bigger the show of force, the more the crowd gathers. Sometimes going in quietly is the safest way to get in and out of these situations without getting into trouble.

As we got closer, we recognized the victim on the ground: Wheelchair Willie. We knew him very well. We treated him for something a couple of times a month. He was a local resident, a drug dealer. He got his chair about five years earlier because of a gunfight with another drug dealer over turf.

We began to assess our patient and things were not good. Willie was definitely going to die and there was nothing we could do about it except make it look as if he had a chance. People in the project didn't trust authority figures. They didn't trust the police, they didn't trust firefighters, and they didn't even trust the "street doctors," as paramedics were called, especially white ones. All of the responders on this call fell into that category. We had to hurry. Any perception by the crowd that we white folks were not doing our job right would lead to violence against us. Fresh in our memories was an incident involving one of our coworkers who had been assaulted a week earlier, just down the street. She was punched in the face and shoved down a flight of stairs by a relative who was unhappy with the speed of care being rendered to his mother. I looked up and noticed the cop looking more nervous with each passing second. His eyes were darting over the crowd, looking for any sign that the shooter was watching, waiting to see if Willie needed to be shot a few more times to finish the job.

As we worked on him, bent over in the rain, I heard a shrill voice through the bedlam. "Doctor, you going to save his ass or what?" I knew the voice without even looking up. It was Willie's lady, Darlene. They made quite a team. She was a ninety-pound, sickly-looking addict who lived with Willie. She got drugs, and Willie got help to and from his chair and the money from Darlene's side business as a hooker.

"Darlene, we're going to do our best." I lied. "He's hurt really bad this time."

Now the screaming ratcheted up a notch from the crowd, most of whom were members of Willie's customer base. John and I made eye contact and our look said it all, *Put on the show for the crowd, get Willie in the ambulance, and get out of here before he dies.*

There were three bullet holes in his chest, two in his abdomen, and two more in his useless legs. Willie was so badly injured that he'd stopped bleeding, which is always a bad sign. We put the oxygen mask in place and applied the cardiac monitor leads, which showed a completely lethal heart rhythm. Willie's body was secured to a backboard with two straps, and we headed for the ambulance. The cop provided a very false sense of security for us, and the crowd surrounded us and followed us like a premature funeral procession.

We loaded the stretcher. John hopped in and began to listen to the fading sound of Willie's heartbeats. He hung a 1,000cc bag of IV solution as the crowd watched the show. I closed the door, got in the driver's seat, shook my head at the cop, indicating the outcome, and completed the final act of our street play by flipping on the lights and siren, leaving the project as fast as I could get us out of there. I looked in the mirror to see the cop following me, adding to the show with his lights on as well. The noisy parade was all part of an illusion created to allow us to say that we had done all we could. It would allow us to face these same people on the same street tomorrow and not get hurt for not saving Willie.

We arrived at the hospital three very short minutes later. The IV was running and Willie's veins were so depleted of blood that there wasn't going to be any catching up. John was sweaty from doing three minutes of CPR. The trauma team stood at the door of the ambulance. We pulled the stretcher from the rig and gave a report. The doctor looked at Willie's wounds, listened to his heart, and pronounced Willie dead with a simple statement: "Time of death 23:13." We never even made it into the ER. We were still on the ambulance ramp.

The doctor looked at us and said, "Nice job, guys. How'd you even get a line on him?"

John wiped his face and said, "I dug."

The head nurse, Greg, looked at me and said, "Sorry, guys. We're swamped. You've got to take him to the morgue for us. I'll get the key and a toe tag and take you down there."

Just like that, Wheelchair Willie and his business enterprise ceased to exist, all in twenty minutes from the first report of the shooting to the presumption of death.

Four other things also happened in that same twenty minutes: Someone took over Willie's business territory; someone was planning retaliation for the shooting; Darlene would be working for somebody else by midnight; and a shooter was still loose in the north end of Hartford.

We cleaned up the truck after the morgue visit and John said, "I'm starving. How about a slice from that place down by the train station?"

"Sounds good to me."

I took a left out of the ER parking lot, heading downtown. So far, it was a normal Saturday night, and we were only four hours into the twelve-hour shift.

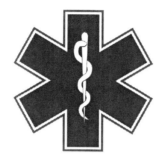

CHAPTER 10

A SHIFT FROM HELL

A SHIFT FROM HELL

It was New Year's Eve 1986 and we'd been on the street as newly minted medics since May. We'd gotten a lot of life saving under our belts, and we were ready for whatever the night might throw at us. New Year's Eve had always been what I called rookie night, when unpracticed drinkers headed out on the town and then tried to get home again. The night was either quiet or insane; there was no in between. For years I'd always volunteered for this shift because the entertainment was the best in town. I was usually paid overtime to hold down a front row seat, except that now, because I was managing the company, there was no overtime for me. I'd been looking forward to this shift. My partner, who also volunteered for the night, was a hilarious guy named Jeff. He was a gangly 6'1", weighing about 130 pounds when soaking wet, and he was known far and wide for the Maglight™ that he carried, a monstrous eight-D-cell, aluminum flashlight that looked like a softball bat. The thing had to weigh ten pounds, and he claimed that he carried it "purely because it gives better light."

Bullshit. I think it's part self-defense and part an anchor in case the wind kicks up. It'll hold him down.

We checked out the rig and I started to overstock the supplies. How many bandages? How many oxygen masks? How many cervical collars? I was insuring that the basic stock was there and then adding to it.

Jeff looked at me in a weird way, and cocked his head to the side. "What are you doing?"

"I've got a feeling."

He shook his head and started walking away. He hadn't gotten ten feet from the ambulance when the radio squawked, "453," our unit designation. "Priority one, Albany and Vine for a man down. Nothing further. Multiple calls." We just looked at each other, hit the lights, hit the siren, and headed off, knowing a couple of things.

First of all, a simple man-down call never gets multiple calls. Most people simply step over the body. They assume the guy's lying on the ground drunk, and they just keep moving on, so I just knew for a fact this one was going to be work.

Jeff was also notorious for one other thing besides his flashlight: his driving. I wasn't actually sure if we were in an ambulance or a rocket sled. All I could do was hang on and hope I was going to survive getting to the call because he was weaving in and out of traffic at a very high rate of speed.

We arrived to find what we in the business affectionately called the "uh-oh squad" gathered around the body of a man lying face down on the sidewalk.

The uh-oh squad is the group of people that seem to gather at every type of incident to rubberneck and say, "Uh-oh. What happened? Ooh. Ah. What's going on?" They typically get in the way and provide an uninvited audience for whatever it is that we do, watching our every move and comparing it to what they see on TV.

The uh-oh squad parted for us, revealing the guy lying face down on the sidewalk. All around him I could see moisture in the glow of the streetlight—a lot of it. As we approached, I could see and smell that the liquid on the ground was a mixture of booze from the broken bottle that he'd dropped next to him and blood.

I took hold of his head to protect his neck and we prepared to log-roll him over. In case he had a spinal injury, we kept his spine straight, but we needed to get him from his stomach onto his back so we could see what was going on. We wanted to see where the blood was coming from because nothing was visible on his back. As we got ready to roll him over, I fully expected to see a head laceration, because even when head lacerations are not that serious, they bleed a lot. Neither Jeff nor I were prepared for what we saw when we rolled him over: his abdomen was sliced completely open and his intestines were exposed, which, in technical terms, is called an evisceration. The stereo "Holy shit!" that came from both of us as well as the bystanders would have been funny under other circumstances.

We had to really move quickly to save this guy. Jeff ran for a device called the scoop stretcher, a metal device that splits apart so you can slide it under victims and scoop them up from underneath. It makes moving people easier than a backboard in some circumstances.

I still held the man's head and I assessed the damage from my vantage point, looking down from his head. At this point, the uh-oh squad started to leave.

"That's disgusting. I got to go."

"Holy crap," or "That's just sick."

One guy looks queasy.

Go away! I really don't need another patient right now.

Jeff came back with the scoop and a collar. We quickly put the collar on the man, got him into the scoop, strapped him down, and got him into the truck.

Nobody in class told me how much blood and guts stink.

His abdomen was cut from side to side, completely open. Once in the truck under the bright fluorescent overhead lights, I could see the true extent of the damage. This guy was almost sliced in half at the waist. None of the bandages we had in the truck were going to be adequate to cover him up, even if I emptied the overstocked cabinet. The trauma dressings just weren't big enough. I had no choice, so I opted for sheets.

What the hell? It's three minutes to the hospital and I'm not going to have to look at it anymore. That'll work out really well.

Jeff started the drive to the hospital. I put on a nonrebreather mask, which is a green plastic oxygen mask with a little clear plastic bag at the bottom that gives the patient the highest concentration of oxygen possible short of intubating him. He needed as much oxygen as possible in his bloodstream because he was losing blood very fast. It was three minutes to the hospital, so I had to work fast. I started two large-bore IVs, one in each arm, and connected each to a 1,000 cc bag of fluid. Once they were in, I just kept squeezing them, trying to get as much fluid into him as quickly as possible. I put the heart monitor on and looked at the heart rate; it was fast but not lethal. Jeff made a turn and said, "We're here."

We pulled the stretcher out, bringing it up to height, and ran into the emergency department to face a very surprised triage nurse. In the hurry to do all of this, we forgot to call the hospital to say we were coming. She had no idea that we were pulling in with a life-threatening case.

"Hi, Marge. Forgot to call. Evisceration. Trauma room. Now," I called over my shoulder as we kept walking by her to our destination, the trauma room. Hopefully there was an open bed there.

I knew I was going to get my butt reamed out later for not giving them a heads-up, but, hey, I was working.

The entire trauma team began to assemble; the surgeons arrived, anesthesiology came in case they had to put him out, and they started to do their magic. I turned the patient over to them and said, "I don't know anything more. He was found face down. There's alcohol involved somehow or he dropped the bottle. I don't know which. Do a blood alcohol level," which they're going to do anyway. "We were three minutes from here. You saw what I got. I got the monitor on. I got two lines, oxygen, and then we were here."

I wanted to stay and watch, but Jeff came running back in. "Hey. We've got to go. They've got an MVA with entrapment down the street and we're it."

I started to protest, but I realized if they're sending *us* to this call, knowing what we had just brought in, the other eight ambulances that were on duty were already on calls.

Good thing I thought to stock up.

This call was literally a mile from the hospital. With my NASA-trained pilot, we arrive in under a minute. The carnage was impressive. The car, which was a full-sized 1980-era sedan, had struck the side of a concrete bridge, head on. The road curved at this particular point and apparently the driver had missed that part of the navigation class. This was in the days before antilock brakes were invented, so we were able to tell there were no skid marks, which meant it was a full speed impact.

Through the windshield we could see what was left of the front end of the car. We were trying to calculate where the engine was. Jeff, ever helpful, said, "With that much damage, the driver and the engine block ought to be in the back seat."

We pulled up, got out, approached the car, and reported to the captain of the fire department's rescue squad. He looked past me at the single ambulance and said, "You got more units coming?"

"Nope. We're it for now. What do you got?"

"There's two obvious dead, three critical. They're all wedged in the back seat by the engine block and the front of the car."

I looked back at Jeff, who shrugged.

I told you so.

"Can I get to access any of them, Cap?"

"Yeah. We popped the rear passenger door, and as long as you're okay around the cutters, you can get in there. We'll just cover you up with the tarp while we cut."

I grabbed a flashlight, the monitor, and IV bag, and I headed into the back seat and climbed under the tarp.

This is what a dead guy feels like. I don't want to join them because I can't see anything going on outside while I'm under this tarp.

Jeff's job was to stand guard outside the door, protect me, hand me stuff, and remind the fire guys that there was a medic in the back seat while I was doing what I was doing.

Now I was under this tarp. A quick look around with the flashlight revealed two males and a female all in their early twenties. Both males were unconscious. The woman was semiconscious, moaning in pain, the engine block sitting squarely on both of her legs, which are clearly broken in multiple places.

They better cut fast or we're going to lose all of them.

I was very familiar with the Jaws of Life, the heavy hydraulic spreader cutters that are used to separate cars from people, but I'd always been on the other side of this situation in heavy firefighter turnout gear. This was a first, being under a tarp, working by flashlight, listening to the grinding and the tearing and the tortured shriek of the metal that they were cutting.

No wonder patients are scared when we're doing this.

From where I was, I could only get to the guy that was closest to me. I could reach across him to get to the girl, but I had no way to reach the other passenger. I could see and hear his labored breathing, but triage rules applied, and I couldn't treat everybody. He was going to have to be left on his own until we had either more room or more people. The girl got oxygen first. She was clearly more critical with her injuries and loss of blood. Soon enough I got oxygen for the guy as well, because the firefighters gave us their bottle off the rescue truck. I could get to one arm on each of them, so I put large-bore IVs in both of them.

I yelled to Jeff, "Go get more bags of IV fluid, because these are going to empty quick."

I heard a loud groan, muffled voices, and someone yelling, "One, two, three." I heard what sounded like rain on the tarp, and all of a sudden it became noticeably cooler under there. I realized they'd finished cutting and they'd pulled back the roof. The rain sound was made by small little kernels of windshield and window glass that were now everywhere. I realized we were going to have to be careful or we'd all get cut up, because the minute they moved this tarp, if they didn't move it just right, glass would rain all over me and my patients.

They did a great job of removing the tarp, but as they removed it, I was momentarily blinded by the big spotlights on the top of the rescue truck. I heard sirens in the background, and Jeff's voice. "What do you need? 462 just arrived and 451 is three minutes out." Two more ambulances. Reinforcements were coming.

"Hey, Cap, how much longer?" I yelled.

"We'll have access to the guy you haven't treated first. The girl is going to be last."

They had popped a door and taken it off, courtesy of the cutters, so the other ambulance crew could reach the injured man I couldn't get to.

Now that I had better access and light, I could prepare my two for extraction. The guy was going to go next. The firefighters setup a hydraulic ram, because they needed to lift part of the metal off him. He was trapped by crumpled sheet metal and seats, but they'd need the ram to get my girl out anyway, because they had to move the engine block.

The lead fireman said, "Hey, medic, you need to clear for a minute. We can't get around you."

I didn't want to leave, but I saw his point. I was in their way. I told both patients, whether they could hear me or not, "I'll be right back."

The girl was whimpering. The guy was still out, but I hoped he heard me.

The Hartford Fire Department rescue guys were really good. They made short work of the pile of scrap metal, and I returned with Jeff and the other ambulance crew. They'd take the guy. I'd stay with the girl until she was out. They got the guy boarded and out of the way, and now I had even more space in which to work and take care of her. I had my doubts about her survival. It had been forty-five minutes now, and she was losing consciousness and going into shock. I'd done what I could. She was on oxygen. I ran a third bag of IV fluid into her veins. My real fear was that when they lifted the engine block off her, she'd hemorrhage massively, and she'd die right there in the car.

I told the firefighters and Jeff, "Listen. We're going to slide the backboard in behind her. As soon as her legs are clear, we're coming straight up the backboard and then we're going to tilt her onto the back of the trunk. Manage her neck, C-spine control. Don't worry about her legs, no matter what shape they're in. Just worry about her head and her torso." I worried that when we tried to move her, something would be disconnected; in fact, I expected it. Her legs were so massively fractured that it seemed likely that not all of her body parts would come with her when we moved her. I still had no idea what her name was. I said, "Listen. We're going to get you out, but it's going to hurt like hell and we really have no choice."

I looked to the firefighter who controlled the ram and nodded. Everybody was in place. The valve opened, the ram pushed, the engine moved very slightly, and the girl came out of her semiconscious state and screamed. We had no choice; we had to continue. Finally we got enough clearance to free her legs and as we slid her up the board, we had almost everything, except her left foot. The rest of the crew strapped her to the board and moved her to my ambulance. I reached under the engine, hoping that the ram would hold, and I found her foot.

Nice high heel. We should bring this just in case they can save it.

I took it and went.

The ride back to the trauma room was, again, a minute longer than the flight down there. I looked at my watch, sixty-two minutes since the time of call. We had two dead, three critical so far, and the night was still young. We arrived at the hospital, where they were already tired of seeing us because we'd just brought in the evisceration. We learned that our evisceration guy had got in a fight over his bottle of booze. He'd pulled a knife, but his attacker had pulled a machete. He was barely alive. We put the truck back together and grabbed a lousy cup of ED coffee. Jeff glared at me, at this point, through the coffee steam.

"What?" I ask with a grin on my face.

"You and your feelings."

I held my coffee cup to my head, like a fortune teller, "I feel… like a cardiac arrest."

"Great," was all he said, and he walked away, shaking his head.

Note:

The shift was thirteen hours long and Jeff and I ended up doing twenty-two calls, with a total of five fatalities. It was the single busiest shift of my career.

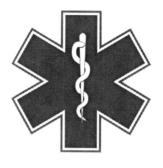

CHAPTER 11

MANAGEMENT:
A NEW KIND OF STRESS

MANAGEMENT: A NEW KIND OF STRESS

When I left the Corrections Department and finished paramedic school, I accepted a job as the general manager of the ambulance company. So I was not only pulling shifts for fun and excitement, learning how to be a good paramedic, but I was also managing a staff of about 125 people, doing scheduling, and making sure the trucks were maintained. I had the responsibility to make sure that the crews were doing their paperwork properly, so we could bill the calls out and get paid. I only worked one job, but I was still working about ninety hours a week. The bad part of this was that instead of being on a shift for twelve hours, then getting off and going home, now I was on call twenty-four hours a day. I had a pager. I had a radio in my car to talk to dispatch. I had lights and a siren in my car in case I needed to get some place as the chief of service.

If something went wrong, if an ambulance got in an accident, if there was a major incident or something that the shift supervisor couldn't handle, they bumped it up to me. It could be two in the morning and a nursing supervisor could be aggravated because of something that happened on a call, and my pager would go off.

I still hadn't realized that down time was beneficial. I hadn't taken time off, other than a long weekend, in probably two years. Between training, school, work, shifts, clinical, and now being out on the road trying to hone my skills, I was taking as many shifts as I could. I dated here and there, and I also had friends and family aggravated with me.

Light dawns slowly on a thick-headed Irishman. I didn't have a serious relationship. I was seeing someone on a regular basis, but typically when we started to get into "that conversation" about where things might go, the pager went off and I had to leave.

My family was frustrated because I'd make a commitment to go to somebody's birthday party, and then we'd have a shift problem and I couldn't go. I was supposed to attend a friend's wedding, and I had to cancel out the morning of the wedding. I couldn't go. I was all wrapped up in running the company. I was twenty-six years old, and it still hadn't dawned on me that this was not really all that healthy. I was in the middle of it.

It was what it was and I was doing a lot of "Sorry, but..." conversations: "Can't go to dinner tonight." "Can't go away for the weekend." "Sorry, I can't make the wedding because we have three ambulances down and I need to be here." It took a couple of years of this, with people saying, "Wake up, will you? We haven't seen you in a year."

I'd make it for Christmas. I'd make it for Thanksgiving, but I might not remember it was somebody's birthday until two days later. Periodically I'd have company over for an evening, but, for the most part, life was get up, go to work, come home, go to sleep.

I realized I hadn't been on a real vacation in awhile, just a few days here and there.

I finally went into the weekly management meeting and announced, "I'm taking a week off."

There was dead silence in the room and then, "You're doing what?"

"I'm taking a week. I'm going on a cruise."

"When are you leaving?"

"Thirty days, I'm leaving. My pager is going to be on my desk. If you set it off, it's going to vibrate off my desk, so you guys are going to have to figure out how to deal with everything for a week without calling me. You might as well get used to it now."

I look back on those years and I don't know what the hell I was thinking, to be honest with you. I would never do that again, but it got me a lot of experience very quickly. I grabbed an opportunity to run a multimillion dollar company at twenty-six. I had the opportunity to grow the market share of the business and try a lot of different things because I was given almost carte blanche to do whatever I wanted to do to improve the company. Then, to be part of bringing paramedics to and advancing the level of care in Connecticut's capital city for the first time—I couldn't say no to that. I just did it. Everything else was on a back burner. I didn't have a wife. I didn't have kids, so it didn't matter, at least in my head at the time. My life was very lopsided for a long period of time. I'm able to enjoy the benefits of those choices now, but I didn't even see what I was doing to the people around me at the time. The good part was that I made some very good long-lasting friendships during those years, and I'm very appreciative that many of those people are still in my life.

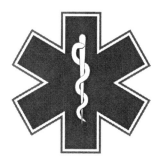

CHAPTER 12

"YOU'RE GONNA CARRY ME!"

"YOU'RE GONNA CARRY ME!"

In Hartford, as in most cities around the country, there is rampant EMS system abuse. The 9-1-1 system is the catch-all service for people who don't have healthcare and for people who don't have transportation. They need to get someplace. They know if they say certain things, ambulances come quickly, and they know that ambulances have to take them where they want to go, within reason. Therefore, the system gets abused.

There's a sort of unwritten EMS rule: the larger the person, the higher up in the building they live. According to the rule, 200-pound people tend to live on the second floor, 300-pound people tend to live on the third floor, and so on. Strange but true; nobody can explain it, but it's a fact.

One night we got a call for a woman who was not feeling well. "Ambulance 451 respond to 206 Main Street, Apartment 3, on the third floor, for a woman not feeling well."

This kind of call is never a good sign because any time the call is nonspecific, you have no idea what you're walking into. It could be nothing. It could be a heart attack. It could be domestic violence.

We carried the gear up and found a lady who weighed about 325 pounds. She was having trouble breathing. She looked at us and said, "You guys need to carry me downstairs. I can't walk."

"Okay. Let's assess you, find out what's going on, and then we'll take good care of you. Don't worry about it."

Something about this lady seemed bogus; patients who have difficulty breathing have a very specific look about them and this woman didn't have it. This seemed more like panting for attention than difficulty breathing. But she was adamant. As we were assessing her, she told me twice again, "I need to be carried."

"We'll get to that. Let's figure out what's going on with you first."

I looked through the apartment for inhalers, for the shoebox full of medications that chronically sick people have. As I looked around, I was struck by the fact that I didn't see a phone. This incident happened long before there were cell phones, so a phone should have been hanging on the wall somewhere and there wasn't one. The woman's name was Martha.

"Martha, how'd you call 9-1-1? Did you call or did somebody call for you?"

"I called."

"Okay. How?"

"I called from my friend's apartment."

"Really? Where's your friend's apartment?"

"On the first floor."

"Let me get this straight. You have trouble breathing and feel that you need to be carried. You live on the third floor. You walked down to the first floor. You called 9-1-1 and then walked back up to the third floor so that we could carry you down."

"Yes."

"All right. That makes no sense to me. Let's continue."

I listened to her lungs, her lungs were clear. I talked to her, and everytime I talked to her, she stopped panting to answer my question, after which she began panting again. I was pretty convinced, and so was Bobby, my partner, that we had a faker on our hands.

"If you walked downstairs to call 9-1-1, you can walk downstairs now, we'll help you."

She started to argue.

"Listen, I'm willing to carry any patient who needs to be carried, but I don't believe you need to be carried. I'm pretty comfortable we can get you downstairs safely, all three of us together. We'll be fine."

She got up, walked across the room, picked up her keys, her cigarettes, and her lighter, walked back, sat down, and said, "Nope. You need to carry me."

Now I was pissed. I'd just about had it. It had been a busy night and this call was bullshit.

I told her, "Ma'am, let me be very precise with you. I don't believe you need to be carried. I don't believe you have any shortness of breath. I think you want a ride to the hospital. I don't know why you want a ride to the hospital, but we're going to give you a ride to the hospital. But I'm *not* carrying you down three flights of stairs when you go up and down the stairs to call 9-1-1, you can walk across the room, and every time I ask you a question, you stop panting. I am not carrying you."

She said, "I am paying for this ambulance trip and you're carrying me."

"All right. I'll play. Ma'am, what type of insurance do you have?" Typically, I wouldn't ask for insurance information—so we can bill for the service—until the call was over, but she had brought up the topic.

She whipped out her Medicaid card. "Right here. My insurance. I'm paying for this trip and you're going to carry me."

"Well, I have good news and bad news. The good news is that you're going to get your ride to the hospital, and I'm going to take good care of you on the way. The bad news is I'm not carrying you because that insurance means I'm paying for the trip, and I'm not carrying your ass down three flights of stairs."

She glared at me. "What is your name?"

"Bob Holdsworth."

"I want the name of your supervisor because I'm calling and filing a complaint against you because if anybody else needed it, you'd carry them. What's his name?"

At this time I was the general manager of the ambulance company, so I said, "Bob Holdsworth."

She glared at me. "I'm filing a complaint with the city."

"The mayor's on my speed dial at my office. We can meet down there if you'd like, but now we're going downstairs. We're going to get in the ambulance. The bus is leaving. You want to go? No more fooling around."

Yes, she wanted to go to the hospital, but not the one three blocks away; she wanted to go to a hospital on the other side of town. We finally walked her down the flights of stairs, and she bitched every step of the way. On the way to the hospital I said, "Just level with me. You're not having trouble breathing and you want to go all the way across town. Why?"

"I have to go visit my sister and she lives down the street from the hospital."

"Okay. I got it." I looked at her. "You could have just said you had to go to Hartford Hospital for a doctor's appointment instead of going through all that garbage. You're a lousy fake. By the way, I am still paying for this trip so have a good day."

This is the kind of stuff that burns EMS people out. I understand that people have economic challenges that they can't get around, that buses don't run after a certain time, and they've got to get some place. They don't know what to do, and 9-1-1 becomes their fallback resource, but it takes the service away from others who really need it.

Had I not been the general manager of the company, I probably would've been the target of a complaint, and more than likely I would have had to deal with a manager saying, "Don't make waves. Next time, carry the person."

It's the abuse and the overuse that kill the spirit. There's nothing more infuriating than getting injured when you are carrying someone who doesn't need to be carried, or getting into a wreck when you are going to something stupid. There's nothing more frustrating than getting to a call only to wonder why you are there.

Seniors tend to use the system most because they live alone, they get nervous, they have a little shortness of breath, and they want someone to come check them out because they don't have family close. For the most part, nobody minds that kind of a call unless it's coming every day. Everyone in this profession wants to take care of that person and say, "We'll check your blood pressure. We'll check your blood sugar. You'll be okay."

It becomes abuse when we are called out to help the same people who keep falling out of bed, because they won't put up a side rail. It's especially aggravating to volunteers who have to get out of bed to go on call. We're the safety net. People know that when you dial 9-1-1 you're going to get an ambulance, you're going to get a cop, or you're going to get a fire truck. By dialing three numbers you're going to get service. The bigger the town, the more delayed the help might be because of prioritization of calls, but eventually somebody's going to come.

With all of the stress, when there's a lull between calls, high-energy people find creative ways to blow off steam. Adrenaline junkies need something to do, and we can get inventive.

One of the pastimes we enjoyed for a short time was munchkin tag. Unbeknownst to most people who think they are merely edible little balls of sugar, munchkins are actually quite aerodynamic, which is why, having nothing much to do between calls except drink coffee, bitch, and find new ways to antagonize management, somebody in our company invented munchkin tag.

The rules of munchkin tag are very simple. You drive around the city looking for other units from your company who are also attempting to find you. The driver pilots the vehicle and the ambulance attendant's job is to launch munchkins at the other truck. The game was to patrol the district and see how many points you could get. Hitting the truck counted as a hit, but not a good one. Hitting the windshield was considered to be a solid kill. Powdered munchkins were the weapons of choice because there was no denying a hit. A glazed munchkin would roll off the windshield. A powdered munchkin would leave a mark. Points were given, and the loser typically had to buy coffee.

The game ended quickly after somebody came up with the idea of upping the stakes by using jelly-filled munchkins. When they hit a windshield and splattered, you had to stop the truck because the windshield wipers will not clean off the jelly effectively. Plus, it looks nasty, which is even more fun—and more dangerous. The game of munchkin tag was ruined by the jelly munchkin.

Blizzards were fun too. In a snowstorm, normally, ambulances should be deployed around the city, but when the storm was really bad, nobody was going anywhere. One particular park had this really nice hill. We took the trucks there, pulled out the backboards, and turned them into toboggans with nine-foot straps.

Three of the six ambulances that were on duty were all in the same spot; six ambulance attendants were dripping wet from sliding down a hill in their uniforms, and the backboards and the straps were now soaked. Other than that, it was a lot of fun.

The ambulances would be brought to the edge of the hill with the white side-lights on, and the spotlights would be pointed down the hill so you could see where you were going. Afterward, we'd go off to warm up at whichever coffee shop was still open.

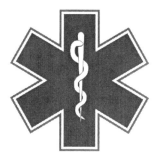

CHAPTER 13

A MOTORCYCLE, A POLICE CAR, AND A CANOE

A MOTORCYCLE, A POLICE CAR, AND A CANOE

On this particular night, I was going to work with a guy who was affectionately known as "Trauma" Tom Higgins (1949–2012). Tom had been around the business for a long time and he and I had gone through both intermediate and paramedic class together. I was the general manager of the ambulance company, and he was one of my supervisors, so we never worked together, but there just happened to be an opening because his usual partner banged out sick.

I decided that would be a good time to jump in and do a night shift, just to see how the other half lived, because administrators were always around during the day. Tom was notorious for having a cigarette and a cup of coffee in one hand at all times. We were going to go grab some food, so we pulled into the Burger King drive-through. We were just getting our food when the radio crackled: "451, New Park Avenue, West Hartford near our old office, car versus motorcycle."

We took off. The lights were on; the siren was going; Tom was driving. Tom had his usual cigarette and coffee in one hand and the burger from Burger King in the other. We rocketed down Prospect Avenue and I tried to figure out exactly what he was driving with, because both of his hands were already occupied.

As we responded, we received more information from the dispatcher. "Be advised, we're not sure exactly what's happening, but there's a police officer involved in the accident." So now we were not sure whether a motorcycle cop had been injured, or whether a police cruiser had been in a collision with a motorcycle, and we were already going as fast as the truck would go. I was really concerned that Tom was driving with his knee and we were doing about ninety miles an hour down the street.

More from the dispatcher. "We're getting multiple calls from the police department; you need to expedite."

"Expedite? The truck doesn't go any faster, I don't know what you want me to do," I yell back into the radio. As we turn the corner and come onto a straight part of the road, we could see the police cruiser with its lights on, about a half-mile ahead of us, and we got the last update that the accident was the result of a police chase and they weren't sure who was hurt.

I grabbed the microphone. "We'll be there in thirty seconds. We'll let you know."

Arriving to a very pungent smell of burning brakes, we saw a car and the cruiser facing each other about twenty feet apart. A motorcycle was wedged underneath the car. A police officer was kneeling in the road over a guy who was obviously the motorcycle rider, pushing down on his legs. That's all we could see, except for the fact that in the middle of all of this, a canoe was sticking out of the windshield of the police cruiser. I looked at Tom and said, "I can't wait. This is going to be a great story."

As we got out, the cop yelled, "Hurry up, he's bleeding!"

I asked Tommy, "What do you want for equipment?"

"Bring everything," he said and took off. His cup of coffee was in the dashboard holder, his cigarette was flung out the side of the truck; he was done with the cheeseburger because he'd inhaled it; and he ran to take care of the patient. I would defer to him because although I was his boss, he had more experience in the field than I did by several years.

We got to the cop. "What happened?"

"I was chasing the guy; he dumped the bike; the bike went under the car; and he stopped here. The car was carrying the canoe and when the bike jammed underneath it, the car stopped, the straps broke, and all I saw was a canoe coming at me. I bailed out of the car and came over here to take care of him."

Good synopsis.

I looked at Tom. "I told you it would be a good story."

The guy lay in a massive pool of blood. The cop said, "His femoral artery is bleeding. I've got my hand on it. If I take my hand off, it's going to squirt like a geyser."

I looked at Tom and said, "I'll get the mast trousers," which are military antishock trousers that you slide on and inflate to apply pressure. They're not used anymore, but at the time they were used by the military and adopted by civilian paramedics to force blood out of the lower extremities back into the core of the body when somebody was severely injured. In this case, this would also put pressure on the femoral wound to stop it from bleeding.

Tom pulled a huge trauma bandage out of his kit and said to the cop, "Go ahead and move your hand." The minute the cop lifted his hand up, blood just sprayed straight up in the air while Tommy was trying to slide the bandage on top of it. By the time I covered the fifteen feet from the truck to hand him the trousers, I could see that the bandage he had just put on was already starting to soak through. We knew that between the blood that was on the ground and the blood that was on the bandage, this guy had probably lost a third of his blood supply. We didn't have a lot of time and we were going to have a lot of making up to do.

We also could see that his other leg was kind of in the shape of a Z, so we knew that it was broken in at least two spots. We didn't know what else had gone on because we hadn't even had time to assess him; we had to control the bleeding first.

We examined him and found he had seven compound fractures, meaning seven different wounds with broken bones visible in them, plus the femoral artery bleed, plus the fact that he'd lost a lot of blood. We tried to figure out where we could put IV's in him because you can't put IV's below a fracture; you have to go above the fracture. Otherwise, you're going to have it run right out through the fracture. Finally we found a couple of spots above the fractures where we could insert IVs, get him on the backboard, and get him in the ambulance.

I took off for the hospital with Tom in the back. Tom had two lines going in him, and we'd got the IV bags under pressure so we could put the fluid into him faster. I drove as fast as I could without bouncing Tom around the back of the ambulance. I called out the turns to him so that he could grab the handrail on the ceiling as if he were riding a subway train and hold himself steady. I gave him the countdown to ED. "We're going to be there in a minute; start getting yourself together." He had to switch the guy from the main oxygen to the portable oxygen to go into the ER. While he'd been treating the patient, I'd picked up the radio and done a med-patch to St. Francis to let them know we were coming in. They were ready for us.

As we turned the guy over to the crew in the trauma room, Tom just looked at me and started laughing.

"What are you laughing about?"

"I've been doing this for a long time and I've never seen a canoe in a cruiser, ever." We found out afterward that the guy survived.

He actually came and found us several months later. He walked into the ambulance building, and we were able to meet him under better circumstances.

I'd taken that night shift with Tom partly just to get out of the office that night, because it was a stressful time; we were short on personnel and long on demands. We had taken on the City of Hartford's police contract a few years before and had to hit target numbers for the medics on the road.

I finally took that week-long cruise vacation, but things hadn't calmed down any when I got back, and I had seven days of digging out to do to get back on track. The stress ratcheted right back up again. I found myself snapping at the staff. I was getting a little bit frazzled, and something inside me said that there had to be something more than this increasingly mundane routine. I knew that something had to change. I either had to find a way to do something new with the ambulance company, or do something else altogether.

It was time for some thoughtful self-assessment. I realized that I was good at operations. I also realized I didn't like operations on a day-to-day basis. I was better at long-term strategic planning and got really frustrated with the day-to-day issues.

Did I need four trucks or five trucks, and the staff whining, "I don't want to work with this one, or that one..." It just drove me crazy. My escape at that point was to grab a couple of buddies and go drinking, or go out and hide in an ambulance and do calls.

The owner of the ambulance company said to me, "I'm thinking of semiretiring in a year or so, and I want you to take over as president of the company."

I don't know if I want to do that.

I agreed to think about it. I looked at the schedule for the next day and evening, and saw that there was an opening on night shift that hadn't been filled.

To hell with the schedule and the paperwork, I'm going to escape and take another night shift.

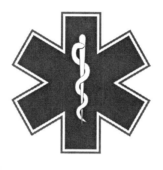

CHAPTER 14

TRAINS AND TRUCKS

TRAINS AND TRUCKS

There's a Dunkin' Donuts on the Hartford/West Hartford line, right around the corner from a three-track, high-speed, railroad crossing. Commuter trains typically go through there at sixty to seventy miles an hour. It was a notorious spot because at least once a year, someone—pedestrian or car—would be struck there. There was a housing project on the other side of the tracks, which created a lot of pedestrian traffic. People didn't understand how fast those trains moved. They'd see the gates coming down, so they'd try to run or drive across the tracks, and they would not make it.

That night, we were in the Dunkin' Donuts parking lot with another truck. We were assigned to the west side of Hartford and the other truck was assigned to West Hartford. We're having coffee when a dispatch came over the radio calling the West Hartford truck: "463, we've got a report of a pedestrian struck; train versus pedestrian." We had just heard the train whistle and the train barreling through the intersection. I looked at my partner. We hadn't done a call all night and these guys had already done a couple of reasonably decent calls.

I said, "We're taking this one."

"The hell you are!"

My partner took his coffee, threw it onto the windshield of the other truck and laughed. "We got it; you seem to be delayed."

We signed on and took off. All we heard were screaming expletives and "We're coming with you!" So lights on, siren on, we turned left out of the parking lot, went 1,000 feet to the intersection, took another left, and came up to the tracks. A cruiser was coming across the tracks from the other direction, and we stopped. The cop was on his radio, calling Amtrak's police dispatcher to tell him that we now had emergency personnel on the tracks, and he should have all the trains coming into this crossing stop or slow down. We all had flashlights, which we waved around to make sure that an approaching train's engineer would see us—at 70 mph. It made us feel better.

One person looked down the tracks for the victim, and the other person's job was to look down the tracks for approaching headlights. We had no way of confirming that the trains had gotten the information. If we had seen a headlight, we would have had a very short amount of time to get the hell off the tracks.

As we started walking, we saw a kid, maybe fifteen or sixteen years old, sitting on the side of the track. He was pure white and shaking. I put my hand on his shoulder, "What happened?"

"Man, we were just walking across the tracks and he went running across, never saw the train. I'm pretty sure he got hit by the train, because I don't know where he is."

"Okay. Okay. We'll go look."

There are only a few possible things that can happen to pedestrians who are hit by trains at seventy miles per hour: they're either going to literally explode—train engineers refer to it as "red mist" when they hit an animal or hit a person at that speed—or they're going to get smacked by the train and may get pulled under it, or they may get tiddly-winked off the side of the train, and they're going to be down an embankment or up in a tree. There may be pieces missing.

We knew which way the train was going because we got the kid to point. So we knew that we needed to look on both sides of the tracks and we needed to look several hundred yards down the tracks, because we didn't know how far the body might have flown. We needed to look up in the tree branches and we needed to look down in the gully beside the tracks to see if we could find this kid. We were prepared to find a severely injured kid, a dead body, or remnants, as we walked. Additional police officers showed up, and our other crew showed up after quickly washing their windshield so they could see where they were going.

"What do you want us to do?"

"Pick one side of the tracks, walk down, and look for any evidence." We all fanned out with our flashlights, and searched the ground. It was pitch black and everybody was watching to be sure a train wasn't coming. As we got about seventy-five or eighty yards down from where the kid said he had last seen his buddy, we found a leg. Clearly this was not going to end well.

We heard a member of the other crew on the other side of the tracks say, "I've got an arm."

The Amtrak police now had a very extended crime scene. They had to reconstruct all of this.

As we kept walking, we found the torso of this kid, and the torso had the other arm attached, so we had that part. We walked down a little further and we found a leg. Interestingly enough, the leg had a *different* shoe. The first leg we found had a black shoe and this one had a red sneaker. We walked down a little bit further because we still had some pieces missing from the puzzle—and we found another torso. We had two victims.

I sent the cop back to ask the kid how many kids were with him.

Two. The kid had assumed the other boy had made it across the tracks, but apparently they had both been clobbered. After about twenty minutes we found all the body parts except for one. A head was missing.

I turned to the Amtrak cops. "Did your dispatcher stop the train?"

"Yeah, it's at Hartford station."

"Ask them to look." And there, on the front of that train, they found the missing head.

My partner, always the optimist, said, "I guess it's a good thing the head stayed on the train."

"It's a *good* thing?"

"Yes, could you imagine that falling off and Fido picking it up and bringing it home to his owner? We would have had a chest pain call."

You never know what to expect. You pull into what you think is going to be one kind of call and it turns into something very different. This call was one that could have ended a lot of careers. People in this business burn out in ten years, and some a lot sooner. Some people have that first absolutely critical call early on in their career and they never make it past that; some people don't get it until they've been at it for fifteen years.

Because of where we worked, we got a lot of critical, ugly calls, one after another. You have to learn how to compartmentalize things; it's simply self-defense.

The bad part of that is that you compartmentalize things at work but you also compartmentalize when you go home. That's why there's so much emotional disconnect among people in the profession. It's taken me a long time to be able let my emotional side re-emerge.

A couple of weeks later, working with a different partner, I was called out onto the interstate for a car versus tractor-trailer. It was a rainy night and the area of the interstate that we were called to was notorious for crashes. We figured it was going to be work. Dave drove way too fast, weaving in and out of traffic. I said, "You do realize how big this truck is, right?"

He looked at me with this absolutely straight face, and said in a deadly serious voice, "You know the faster we go, the thinner it gets, right?" And he shot between two cars with so little room to spare that I honestly didn't know how we didn't hit one of them. We got out onto the highway and could see the cruiser lights way up ahead.

We were about a quarter-mile from the scene and driving over, around, and through car parts—glass, door handles, bits of metal, bits of bumper—not good. We pulled up and saw a car but no tractor-trailer.

I got out and asked the trooper, "I thought this was a car versus tractor-trailer?"

"It is. I'll tell you the story in a minute." He answered his radio.

The trailer portion of the tractor-trailer had gone over the back of this little Ford Fiesta. There was not a piece of glass left in this car and you could see where the wheels of the truck had gone over the hatchback just behind the driver's door. The roof was crushed and the driver was still sitting in the car. We expected this guy to be mangled. We walked up and looked at him. He just sat there, slumped over.

"Hey man, you all right?" Dave asked as he reached in to stop the guy's neck from moving.

The guy answered, in his best '70s hippie voice, "That was amazing."

"Crap, he's *conscious*," I said, looking at Dave. "Buddy, are you okay?"

"Dude, my arm hurts."

"Okay. Anything else?"

"No, man. The trooper dude just told me to sit here and wait for you all."

"You want to tell me what happened?"

"I was driving down the road, and I started to spin around, and I saw the headlights, and then I heard a crunch, and then I saw a tire, and then I bounced off the guardrail like a Ping-Pong ball, and then I just stopped here."

"Have you been drinking?"

"No, dude. I don't drink."

"Do anything else?"

"Oh yeah, some good shit."

"We're going to put you on the backboard, and we're going to put a collar on you and go get some X-rays."

We got him backboarded and bandaged. He said his neck didn't hurt, and his back didn't hurt, but he was high so we couldn't take any chances. We were going to take precautions anyway.

We got him in the ambulance and I went over to the trooper. "What the hell happened?" I asked. "I thought it was a tractor-trailer."

"It was. We stopped it in Rocky Hill," which is four towns down the highway. "He's on his way back. That guy over there," and he pointed to another car parked on the road, "saw the accident and called it in. We had to pull the truck driver over and tell him he had to come back to the scene of the accident. He didn't know he'd been in one, just thought he'd hit some debris on the road."

We took "Dude" to the hospital and "Dude" ended up with a couple of lacerations that did not need sutures, and a broken right wrist. And that was it. Lucky dude. You just never know what to expect.

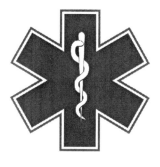

CHAPTER 15

TIME FOR A CHANGE...AGAIN

TIME FOR A CHANGE...AGAIN

In late 1986, when I was running the L & M Ambulance Company, I saw a newspaper advertisement for the position of EMS Coordinator at a hospital down in New London—Lawrence & Memorial (L & M) Hospital. I went down and interviewed for the job. Part of the job was to serve as advanced cardiac life-support coordinator, managing all of the ACLS training for the hospital. The program was designed as standardized training for all the nurses and doctors so that everyone could manage cardiac arrests in the same way, as a team.

A committee had also been formed, made up of local fire department and ambulance personnel, who had recognized that there was a need for paramedics in the region. The closest paramedics to New London worked for a private ambulance service in Norwich, about fifteen miles away. It logically fell to the hospital to take on this project to improve emergency medical care in the region.

Despite the fact that he'd hoped I'd step into his job, my boss at the ambulance company in Hartford was tremendously supportive and gave me a glowing recommendation. I was hired, and in February 1987 I left the ambulance company and became the hospital's first EMS Coordinator, taking on the responsibility of building a regional, hospital-based, paramedic program. The committee members studying the issue were really good people to work with. All of the area fire departments and ambulance services were represented on the committee and were working their way through different options when I arrived. They were all very passionate about getting a program started and told me, "You've done this before; tell us what you think ought to be done and we'll work with you."

I spent a year running to city council meetings, meetings of the ambulance service board of directors, and ambulance membership meetings in eleven different towns, to convince them all of the need for paramedics, how prehospital care could be improved, and how we'd work with them, all while getting the hospital to sign off on spending the money for the program. I needed close to half a million dollars to run this regional program. There was plenty of anxiety about how the medics would work with the existing services and enough controversy to go around, but we finally hammered out a great plan.

We managed to get all the endorsements and the state certifications, but we had a problem: I had no formal department budget. The hospital had not given us a budget to buy trucks and equipment and cover payroll.

The director of the emergency department, Dr. Engleke, and a senior vice president of the hospital both believed in the program. We ended up buying the first truck in the way that Radar did in the *M*A*S*H* episode when he shipped the Jeep home in parts. We had monitors coming from one department, and airway equipment coming from another department's budget. The head of purchasing never knew where it was coming from until it was assembled and in the driveway. The medics were all hired as ACLS instructors under my department.

The girl I was dating at the time worked in the hospital's PR department and she and her boss had logos designed for us. We announced a dedication and a start date. By then, the momentum and positive PR we were getting in the papers swung the administration behind us, and we got everything we needed, as an officially sanctioned hospital department.

In March 1988 we rolled into service for first time, and we started responding within the eleven-town region around New London. Seeing the culmination of the year-long project was a great feeling for all of us involved.

Initially, the nursing staff wasn't overly supportive of these new people coming into *their* hospital and doing things without doctors' orders. Paramedics had standing orders and protocols for the treatment of patients, and nurses had very few. Today we have a great relationship with them, but the program's first couple of months saw very, very rocky relations between the medics and the nurses.

The program is coming up on twenty-five years in operation. The staff have responded to almost 400,000 calls, built a great reputation in the region, and have been credited with thousands of lives saved. I am very proud to have had a part in the system's creation.

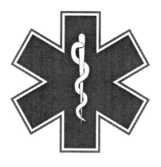

CHAPTER 16

FLYING MOTORCYCLIST

FLYING MOTORCYCLIST

During the year that we were getting the medic program up and running, I had no way to put in any clinical time as a paramedic. I switched to another company in Hartford and worked as a staff paramedic, either at night or on the weekends because I worked at the hospital during the day. I would go down to New London and work all day, and then I would commute back up to the Hartford area and do a twelve-hour shift on the ambulance, just because I wanted to keep my skills up.

I worked for a company called Aetna Ambulance, a company run by two elderly black women. The ambulance company had been around for about forty-five years and had been started by two brothers who married two sisters. The brothers ran the ambulance company and the sisters ran a florist shop downstairs. When the brothers passed away, the sisters ran the florist shop and the ambulance. They were just absolute sweethearts, so much fun to be around.

I said I would work a day shift on a weekend, and was assigned to the medic ambulance in one of the neighboring towns around Hartford. About an hour into the shift we got a call for a motorcycle accident. We ended up getting two ambulances assigned to the call because they weren't sure how severe it was and how many victims were involved. We arrived within a minute of each other, coming onto the scene from opposite directions. A cruiser and a fire engine were already on the scene. In the middle of the road lying on its side, riderless, was what we affectionately referred to as a crotch rocket, one of those sleek motorcycles that can go 150 or 160 mph.

The cop told us that one of the bystanders saw the motorcycle go by, doing seventy-five to eighty miles an hour. Then they heard the screech and the crash. We started to look for the victim. We found a foot, right next to the bike, but no guy. There was nobody there. There were no bushes, no sidewalks, just a bike that had obviously slid a fair distance, and there was a foot on the ground. We looked around, and as stupid as it sounds, we couldn't figure out where the rest of him was. Was there a blood trail? Did he hop away?

Suddenly I heard, "Holy shit!" from John, one of the guys on our other ambulance crew. We all turned to look to see where he was looking. About a hundred feet off the road was a big New England-style house with a white, front-porch railing with the little balusters every three or four inches, and in the middle of this front porch, in the middle of the railing, through the balusters, a body stuck out. The only way that the motorcyclist could have done this was by making a perfect arch through the air from where he dumped the bike. We looked more closely and could actually see broken branches where he had flown through a tree and ended up angling himself right into the railing of this porch with his legs sticking out.

"Holy crap." I grab all the gear and run over to extricate him.

He was unconscious, barely breathing, with multiple fractures, and no helmet of course.

As we put him on the backboard and pulled him out, one of the firemen told us he had called for the helicopter from Hartford, which would arrive in less than ten minutes.

"One problem," he said. "Where do you want me to land it?"

The street we were on was tree lined; the helicopter needed an open area.

The police officer said, "The next street down is a cul-de-sac. Tell 'em to land there."

Great!

"Okay, guys, let's put him in the ambulance, drive him down the street, and we'll meet them there and load him into the helicopter."

We got in the back of the ambulance, and we started working on him, getting him on oxygen, on the cardiac monitor, and putting IVs in him. He stopped breathing, so now I pulled out the laryngoscope, slid the blade into his mouth, cleared the tongue to the left, and the light showed me a perfect set of vocal cords. The tube slid right in between them.

Whew! It's been about a month since I last did that.

I attached an Ambubag to the top of the tube. My partner taped it in place and I began to pump air into his lungs.

Now that we'd got an airway on the guy, we identified his fractures and protected his neck because he obviously went head first through this railing. We drove to the landing zone, the cul-de-sac that was probably 300 yards down the road from where his bike had crashed. We turned around in somebody's driveway and reversed so that the back doors of the ambulance faced the circular end of the cul-de-sac, where the helicopter was going to land.

The helicopter only needed an area of about 60 x 60 feet. There were no power lines or anything else in the way, so they could land right there. As we stopped the truck, we could hear them overhead as they took one pass around the landing area to look for hazards, and then dropped the helicopter right in the middle of the street. As they landed, we kept the doors shut, because the rotor wash was kicking up 120-mile-per-hour wind gusts. We could hear the dust and leaves sandblasting the truck, peppering off the doors.

After about thirty seconds, there was no more sand because they'd cleaned the street, and blown it all on the bystanders who came out to watch. We got out; the flight crew came over; we explained what was going on; they brought their stretcher; we moved him over; and we started to carry him to the chopper.

Now, the whole time we were doing this, the pilot's job was to keep everybody away from the back tail rotor of the helicopter, which was still running as was the large overhead rotor. This was a "hot load," meaning they wouldn't shut the helicopter down because they planned to be on the ground less than ten minutes.

The helicopter had two clam-shell doors in the rear that opened up, and we had to duck under the tail of the helicopter and stay away from the tail rotor because it would have decapitated us if we had not been careful. As we came around the back of the helicopter, we could feel the hot air from the jet engines rushing out over our heads.

We loaded the motorcyclist into the helicopter, and just as we did, the other ambulance came around the corner, and one of its crew came running up. "Here take this, take this, *take this*," he said. He handed the motorcyclist's foot to the flight crew. "I don't know if they can reattach it or not, but here."

At this point we heard bystanders screaming. We didn't understand why, but one woman collapsed into the arms of another bystander. "What the hell is going on with her? Let's get him in the helicopter and then we'll figure it out."

As we loaded the patient, the guys from the other crew went over to the woman who was hysterical and begin to assess her. It turned out that, unbeknownst to anybody, we'd landed the helicopter in front of the motorcyclist's house. He had been going up and down the main street in his neighborhood, and the bike had crashed three hundred yards from his street. We had landed the helicopter and put the motorcyclist in it in front of his family. When the crew-member ran up and said, "Here's his foot," the motorcyclist's mother heard him and screamed; she was the one who passed out. The other ambulance crew took her to the hospital just to make sure that she was okay, but she also got VIP lights and siren ride to the hospital so that she'd be there when the helicopter landed. Sadly, her son didn't make it; most trauma victims who go into cardiac arrest don't.

That was not one of our finest hours, but we'd had no idea. If there's a moral to the story for us, it is that you never know who's watching what you're doing. We learned a lesson that day; keep your mouth shut and just do the job.

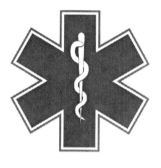

CHAPTER 17

"HIS SOCK IS MOVING"

CHAPTER SEVENTEEN

"HIS SOCK IS MOVING"

During the year that I was working on starting the regional paramedic program, one of the things that I wanted to do was see how other systems worked. I knew how we operated the system in Hartford, and I knew how things had been done in Connecticut by the services providing paramedic service before us. Now I wanted to see how it was done in other places. I started calling up other programs and asking if I could come and visit them and do ride-alongs.

I was looking for the best way to build our system in New London. We were building what's called a paramedic intercept system, designed so that the paramedic is in a separate, nontransporting vehicle and is dispatched to the more serious calls. If they decide the call is not critical, the ambulance transports the patient, and the paramedic unit goes back in service, which means fewer medics can serve a larger area. We had to structure it like that because we were going to be serving eleven towns and about 327 square miles, and we weren't going to have enough paramedics to put them on every ambulance.

One of the arrangements I made was to ride in the City of Boston. I knew the city's paramedics were tied to ambulances, but they were using a district approach that paired basic level and paramedic ambulances on critical calls. I was going to ride for a day, and it was going to be cool for me, because Boston is my hometown.

I arrived at Boston's EMS headquarters, which at that point was an old garage, and I was introduced to Richie, the paramedic I was going to ride with that day. He was washing the truck, having a good time.

"You're awfully chipper for seven in the morning."

He kept washing and said, "A clean truck is a happy truck."

"Okay. You need some help?" He thought it was pretty cool that his rider was going to pitch in and help. It was about 7:10 am when we were dispatched to the Charlestown section of Boston for a reported stabbing.

Richie looked at me. "Stabbing at seven in the morning? This doesn't happen in Charlestown. It has to be you."

Before we could get there, the call was canceled by the other ambulance that had been sent because the wound turned out to be relatively superficial and medics weren't needed.

We got a cup of coffee and started talking. Richie asked me why I was riding, and I told him what we were doing down in Connecticut. He explained Boston's system to me, and we went through the equipment and drugs. He had been with the Boston EMS for quite a long time, so we hit it off pretty well.

About an hour later, we were called to a housing project in Dorchester for a reported man down. We arrived at an eight-story building, a typical, brick, inner-city, project construction. A Boston Housing Authority cop met us there.

"I've got good news and bad news," he said. "The good news is the guy's not in really serious condition."

"Uh-huh."

"Bad news is the elevator's out."

Richie looked at me. "This has to be you."

There were three of us, me, Richie and his partner.

"I'll help you carry him. It's not a big deal." We trucked up seven stories, lugging the oxygen, monitor, drug box, and stair chair. We found this elderly gentleman sitting in a squalid apartment, no air conditioning, and it was hot as hell. The guy wore a grubby T-shirt, hadn't shaved in a while, and sat there in his grungy boxer shorts. We saw the medication vials in a shoebox on the table next to his chair, and we realized that this gentleman was a diabetic. He was not responding properly to us, so we were concerned that his blood sugar was too low. Richie pulled out the glucometer, and began to check the man's glucose. We tried to figure out if he had a blood sugar problem or if he might have had stroke. His vitals were normal, and his pupils were normal, so it was not a stroke. His blood sugar was 42, which is low, but not crazy low. The plan was to put him on the stair chair and carry him down seven flights of stairs in shifts, but it was still going to be miserable. The lucky part was this guy defied the bigger-they-are-the-higher-the-floor rule; he was on the seventh floor, but he only weighed about 140 pounds.

Outstanding.

As we got ready to pick him up and take him from the chair he was sitting on to the stair chair, I looked down, and then tapped Richie on the shoulder.

"Boss, we got an issue."

"Like what?"

"You want to tell me why his sock's moving?"

"*What?*"

"His sock. Is it me, or is his sock moving?" The three of us stood there looking at it, and damned if his sock wasn't moving.

That can't be good.

One of the problems with diabetics is that if they don't take care of themselves, they tend to have circulatory problems, especially in their extremities. When they really don't take care of themselves, these extremities become gangrenous. With gangrene, comes a very particular odor—and maggots.

We looked at each other. Richie said, "I'm not removing the sock. I don't even want to know what's in the sock."

We debated the protocol, because technically there was no injury; the man wasn't bleeding. We had to move him down seven flights of stairs, and somebody had to be at the feet end of the stair chair. If anything happened to this sock, life was going to suck for whoever was carrying the bottom of the stair chair. Clearly we had to find something to cover the guy's foot.

I said, "I got an idea. How about if we take a pillowcase, put the sock and the foot, as is, in the pillowcase, and tape the pillowcase around his leg?"

"Excellent. Like it. Like it."

We found the guy's pillowcase, and then very gently put his foot in it; we didn't want to disturb this sock, because we didn't know how far it was from disintegrating. Ritchie had already put an IV in the guy and given him some glucose, so now he was coming around a little bit, and he was getting a little more anxious, a little more agitated, trying to figure out who we were.

"Hey there; we're from the ambulance. We're going to take you to the hospital."

"I don't really want to go."

"You really need to go. There's something going on with your foot."

He says, "Yes, it's kind of itchy."

Itchy. Right.

"This is *your* fault," Richie said to me.

"I'll take the feet for the first couple floors, then your partner can take over," I said.

It took us about fifteen minutes to carry him down seven flights of stairs. We put him in the ambulance, took him to the hospital, and turned him over to the nurse. I said, "Just be careful of the sock."

"What?" She looked at the pillowcase. "Anyone want to explain *that* to me?"

"Yes, well, there's a surprise in there. He's a diabetic. He doesn't take good care of himself. He has very bad circulation, and his sock was moving."

She says, "Oh, Jesus."

"So, that pillowcase is a safety net. And we're done now. You have a great day."

I had never run into that one before in the field, and especially not on a seven-floor carry down.

Having seen how the Boston system worked, I called a friend who was running University Medical Center's paramedics in Newark, New Jersey. "Can I come down and ride with you guys?" I asked. They also ran ALS ambulances, but they put paramedic supervisors in nontransport vehicles to supervise the system and respond to calls as backup medics. They'd also respond to a need for a medic in one of the surrounding towns. I rode with them for a day, and they just hopped.

Boston was busy, but Newark was like Hartford on steroids. Shootings, stabbings, beatings, car accidents, and drug overdoses; they were getting hammered the day that I went down there. I rode with the supervisor and he showed me the system. There were a couple of nice parts of Newark, but most of the calls were in areas where it wasn't really safe to get out of the truck without a couple of other people around. We worked our way through the day and at about four o'clock in the afternoon we got a call for a possible suicide on a bridge over the highway. Mike, the guy I was working with, said, "We're only a mile away. We'll beat the ambulance in."

"I'll help you," I said. "Tell me what you want me to do and we'll work it out."

We rolled onto the scene, where there were a whole lot more cops than there should have been. Typically in a big city, when there's a suicide, an overdose or something like that, two or three cops show up. If it's a really boring shift, four might show up. As we rolled in, I spotted seven or eight. The fire department and the police shift supervisor were there too.

"This is not going to be normal," Mike said.

We went over to the lieutenant. "What's going on?"

"He's over there." He pointed to the side of the highway overpass we'd stopped on.

"What do you mean? He's *over* where?"

"He's over the edge of the bridge."

Okay. He was over the edge of the bridge. There was a highway below.

"Did he jump already?"

"No, he didn't jump. He's just over there."

Nobody moved really fast. I realized the man threatening suicide was already dead. We went over to look. Hanging by his neck over the edge of the bridge was a male who was obviously dead. His hands were bound behind his back, and his ankles were bound together. This was not a suicide. This was a homicide. This was a crime scene, which explained why everybody was there. The big discussion was about how we were going to cut this 180-pound guy down and get him back over the side of the bridge and back on the street without dropping him onto the highway below. The other question concerned how quickly we could do this, because people were starting to look up and slow down, and we were going to have a traffic collision down below.

A rookie cop came up, looked over the edge, and walked away, shaking his head. He said, "Suicides are so sad, aren't they?"

Everybody stopped dead to see if he was busting our stones or not. Then we realized that he was serious. The whole group just let loose and started laughing. He looked around at us in surprise. "What?"

An officer, who was obviously a veteran, said, "Go look again. Look over the bridge, and tell us what you see."

He looked. Everybody was laughing. The cop finally said. "Oh."
"Yes. Oh."

He had just realized that a suicide can't tie his own hands and feet and then hang himself over a bridge. He had a long way to go to make detective.

The fire department ended up hooking two life belts around the victim so that when they cut the rope they would be able to lift him up and back over the rail. It turned out to be a gang-related murder, intended as a message to a rival gang.

All of this ride-along time was done to fulfill a promise that I had made to my fellow committee members and to all of the agencies in the region: that we were going to design a great system and get the best paramedics available to work with us.

The program we finally launched paired paid paramedics with volunteer drivers whom we solicited from the local EMS agencies. The volunteers learned what the paramedics were about and how we operated. They would drive the medic truck to the scene and back. My philosophy was that if we brought in the local volunteers to work with us, not only would they understand what we did, but they'd become advocates for the program, and volunteers from the smaller, less busy departments would gain experience that would improve their skills.

The system still runs that way, twenty-five years later. In fact, I'm now one of the volunteer drivers. We have an annual volunteer thank-you banquet, and we also started a small fund: for every hour that a volunteer driver works, we put a dollar into an account for them, which they can use for equipment or for education. We've actually put six or seven people through paramedic training, three of whom have gone from being volunteer drivers to being active-duty, paid paramedics with the service.

To make sure we got the best possible paramedics, we used a somewhat unorthodox approach for hiring. We brought them in and sat them down with the head of nursing, the head of the ER, another nurse, and myself. We started with a fifteen-minute oral interview, and then we'd walk them across the hall, and throw them into either a medical or a trauma scenario in which they had to treat a simulated critical patient on the spot. We also put an EMT in the room whose job it was to screw something up while they were running this scenario. We wanted the EMT to either delay doing what he'd been asked to do, or do it wrong. We wanted to see how these potential medic candidates would react to the problem, fix the problem, and educate. We knew we were going to be working with some volunteers who had good skill sets and others who made very few calls a year. We didn't want our medics, as ambassadors for the hospital, jumping down their throats and yelling at them. We wanted them to teach them, and also be able to do great medicine.

When they were done with the scenario, we'd walk them back across to the interview room and interview them for another fifteen minutes. Then we'd send them to a room where they had to document the call—all the drugs that they had given, all the interventions that they had done—to see how good their recollection and documentation skills were. What we ended up with, when we rolled the program out, was a group of great ambassadors who could do medicine. In March 1988, Medic 11 went online in New London, and then a month later Medic 12 went online on the Groton side of the river. Now, we were up to Medic Units 14 and 15, because the volume has exponentially grown over the years.

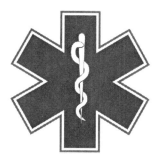

CHAPTER 18

A NEW CHALLENGE: ENTREPRENEURISM

A NEW CHALLENGE: ENTREPRENEURISM

About the same time the paramedic program started in 1988, I hung out my shingle as a consultant, helping the area EMS services. I ran the paramedic program as the EMS coordinator, and I ran my business part-time for a year.

I had spent a lot of time and a lot of emotional energy getting the program established and operating. About a year after the inauguration I again found myself doing operations, not something I was fond of, so I resigned as EMS coordinator, turned the program over to Ron Kersey, who had served as my chief paramedic, and I stayed on for another eighteen years as a staff paramedic.

As I steadily grew my business and traveled all over the United States working with clients, I still worked shifts on a routine basis in New London. Typically, I'd work every Friday, go in at noon and work until midnight or whenever the calls died down. It was not uncommon for me to be by myself on the truck, especially during the first part of the shift.

On this particular morning I came in at 7:00 am rather than at noon, to cover for someone. I checked out the truck, grabbed a cup of coffee, a newspaper, and took the truck down by the water and parked. I rolled the windows down, and sat listening to the ocean and watching the harbor wake up, waiting for whatever the day would bring.

I was less than halfway through my coffee when the tones went off. Each medic unit had a different radio tone, which instantly identified which truck was being sent out. It also alerted other units to listen up in case the call was serious and help might be required.

"Medic 12 respond to South Road for an injured worker…no further details." The address was a cement plant, so this could have been anything from a cut finger to somebody run over by a bulldozer. I was about six minutes away from the scene and making good time moving through morning rush hour traffic. As I drove, I heard a radio call from a fire captain I knew, who had just arrived on the scene. "I need another ambulance. I need another engine. I need heavy rescue, and tell the medics to expedite." This captain, Danny, was highly experienced and a very calm guy. Hearing the decibel level of his voice go up on the radio was enough to make my foot hit the accelerator.

I pulled onto the scene to see his unit, Engine 32, and a second one, Engine 33, already there. Ladder 35, which was carrying some of the heavy equipment, pulled in behind me.

I walked up to Danny. "What have you got?"

"You're not going to believe this."

We were at a cement plant. They had big machinery and big piles of sand. When they opened a door, the sand from the top of the pile was sucked through this machine onto a conveyor belt that carried it up into the plant where it was mixed into cement and ultimately loaded onto trucks. One of the workers, a woman, was up on top of the machine, checking the sand pile for foreign objects, sticks, or whatever. Someone always walked the pile before they turned on the machine.

Danny said, "Somebody accidentally hit the button and turned the machinery on, thinking she was off of it, and she disappeared."

"What do you mean, she disappeared?"

"She got sucked into the hopper."

Holy shit.

"Okay. You got a plan?"

I'm a medic. I know what to do when a patient's available, but I don't know what to do when she's not.

Danny said, "Yes, we're going to start digging from the top and from the bottom. We're going to see if we can get to her from the top, because she couldn't have gone too far, and we'll keep the hopper open in case she comes out the bottom. I want you to stand right here. Don't move, because you can get to her no matter which end we pull her out of."

"How long she's been in there?"

"Well, we got the call the same time you did, and we got here in a minute."

I look at my watch. She'd been in there for about four minutes.

"Okay."

We still had a window of time in which we could save the woman if she were in an air pocket. If she was already in respiratory arrest or cardiac arrest, the clock was ticking. After four minutes without oxygen the body begins to suffer brain damage, and it goes downhill rapidly with every passing minute.

The longer this rescue took, the worse it was going to be. The other complicating factor was that she was in sand, and sand compacts itself around objects, or people. As she was pulled into the sand, the sand would naturally constrict around her, which would make it difficult for her to breathe.

All of the plant's personnel, her coworkers, were on the scene. Everybody was digging, and digging, and digging. I stood there, helpless. I couldn't jump into help, because if I was in the wrong spot when they pulled her out, it wouldn't have done her any good. I just stood there watching those guys and waiting.

All of a sudden I heard someone down below shout, "I got a foot!"

The woman had worked her way through the hopper, which was about ten feet from top to bottom and probably four or five feet wide. They keep digging, digging, digging, and they finally pulled her out and onto the conveyor belt.

I ran to her. She was a small woman. I quickly assessed that she was not breathing.

"Just put her on a board, get two straps on it, and let's get her in the truck. I need light and space."

We had the ambulance crew back their truck up to right where we were, and we loaded her into the vehicle and switched all the lights on.

I had a good crew of folks with me. They were all asking, "What do you want me to do?"

I started assigning tasks.

"I need an airway. You guys get the monitor on. Let's see if we've got a rhythm. Put a tourniquet on each arm so I can get some IVs, and let's get started toward the hospital. Ask dispatch to have Medic 11 meet us en route."

I'm going to need help.

Everyone with me was an EMT. I was the only medic. I had to get an airway. She needed to be intubated. I opened her mouth and found something I was not prepared for. It's not in any of the books. When I opened her mouth, I found it full of sand.

Okay. Think fast.

We had to pull the sand out of her airway, but the suction machine wouldn't do it, because it was designed for fluid.

How am I going to get this out of here? I can't get at her airway, and I can't turn her upside down and just shake her, because she's got to have a neck injury.

I turned to the kid who was in the back with me. "Do me a favor. Hang up one of the big bags of IV fluid and then give me the end of the IV tubing. Turn the main suction unit on and get the portable suction unit too."

"What are you going to do?"

"I'm going to make mud, and we're going to suction it."

"Okay." He sounded skeptical.

"You got a better idea?"

"Hell, no."

"Okay. So let's do this."

We took the IV fluid, 1000 cc of normal saline, opened it up and just let it run, to make mud. We had two suction units going as fast as we could. Every time I made mud, the EMT suctioned it out. We only had to get a baseball-sized amount of sand out, but it took us a minute or two to get it out to the point where I could at least see what I was doing.

"We're going to deal with whatever got into her lungs later, but I've got to get a tube in and start breathing for her."

I removed enough mud to insert a laryngoscope. I could see the vocal cords. I passed the tube, connected the Ambubag, and checked for chest rise and lung sounds to make sure the tube was placed properly.

The lung sounds were diminished.

"They're there, but not great," I told whoever was listening.

"I don't know if she's got chest trauma because she was crushed from the sand."

"Just keep going; bag her; hyperventilate her," which meant squeezing the bag a little faster than normal.

Her pupils were dilated, meaning that she'd been without oxygen for a substantial amount of time, so I knew she'd have some brain problems. She was in cardiac arrest as well, and another guy had been doing CPR on her the whole time we were suctioning out the mud. The monitor didn't show any rhythm at all. That condition is called asystole, meaning there is no electrical activity in the heart.

We just continued CPR. I put an IV in her and pushed epinephrine (adrenaline). I tried to antagonize her heart enough to beat irregularly so that I could defibrillate her. If I could get some electrical activity started, I could send an electrical shock into her heart to jump start it and get it pumping again. It was a long shot, but we had to try because she was just too young.

The ambulance braked hard and stopped.

"Medic 11's here."

The doors opened, and the other medic, Eric, climbed in. I was dripping wet with sweat, and mud was all over the truck. We were doing CPR. I said to him, "You wouldn't believe me if I told you. Just get another line in; push another Epi; make sure we've got good CPR; check the monitor for me. And let's get moving. And somebody call the hospital. Tell them we're coming in with a traumatic cardiac arrest, ETA seven minutes!"

This case wasn't really medically oriented; it was more trauma oriented. We called it that so we'd have the surgeons there if we needed them, and if we didn't, I'd get yelled at later.

The EMT who was working on the woman's chest was doing precision CPR, even though we were in a moving ambulance. The other EMT at the patient's head was hyperventilating her. I watched the monitor, and right after Eric inserted the Epi, I started to see electrical activity.

Ah, it can't be.

So, I told the EMT to stop CPR for a minute. And yes, we had electrical activity. The woman was in a rhythm called ventricular fibrillation (V-Fib), which means the ventricles of the heart are pulsating, wiggling back and forth like a Jell-O mold. This was exactly what I'd hoped for. I could now defibrillate her and hopefully another electrical current was in the muscle fiber of the heart that we could actually get to jump start and fire properly. I told everybody to clear and charged the defibrillator. I got the familiar high-pitched tone. It was ready. I yelled "Clear!" and pushed the button.

The first shock was at 200 joules of current, and her body jerked when it hit her. I looked at the monitor, checked a pulse, wound it up again to 300, got a tone, yelled "Clear!" again, and hit the button. She jumped again, and this time there was a very, very slow heartbeat on the monitor. One of two things was happening: there was either a pulse that corresponded to the heartbeat on the monitor, which meant that the procedure had been successful, or there was electrical activity on the monitor without a corresponding pulse, which was what I expected.

"Check her pulse for me," I said to Eric.

"I've got a pulse."

I didn't believe him. "No, you don't. Get your thumb out of there and check it again."

"No, seriously, no shit. I've got a pulse."

I still didn't believe him, so I put my stethoscope on her chest and I listened to her heartbeat. "No shit. All right. Let's go."

So we had a heartbeat, but we still had dilated pupils and we still had an airway problem. Even though she was intubated, crap obviously remained in her lungs, and she'd been without oxygen for a long time.

We rolled into the hospital. We were turning over a patient we were breathing for, but who had a heartbeat and extremely low blood pressure.

I looked at Eric, and he shook his head. "That was insane. I can't believe we got a pulse back."

"I can't either. I don't even know what to say."

One of the docs came out to talk to us. "Well, she's got a heartbeat, but I don't know how long she's going to keep it."

"Let me know what the EEG shows. I hope she has some brain-function. She was trapped for probably six, seven minutes, and it was at least another two before I could clear the airway, so she was without oxygen for maybe ten minutes."

"You guys did great. We'll see what we can do, and keep you posted."

So, we put the truck back together and went on with our day. Several calls later I was dropping off another patient when the doc told me there was nothing they could do; she had been without oxygen for too long, and she was brain dead. The only saving grace was that her family was able to get to the hospital to spend time with her while she was technically still alive. They signed off on her being an organ donor, and they had plans to donate several body parts.

I went to check on what was going on, and I met her husband. He was obviously devastated, but he said, "I can't thank you enough."

Thank me for what? I couldn't save her.

"The ability for us to be here, and to at least talk to her and say goodbye was priceless. You got her back enough, and she's young enough that she can help ten other people through organ donation. We know that she'll live on through all of those other people, and that's important to us, so thank you."

We were both crying at that point, and I simply hugged him.

You just never know how a call will end. This time, the patient died, but a lot of other people got a chance at life.

Note:

If you have not signed an organ donor card, please talk it over with your family. Tell them your wishes and don't take your organs with you: **www.OrganDonor.gov**.

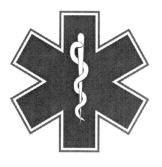

CHAPTER 19

SYLVIA, TOBY AND RESCUE

SYLVIA, TOBY, AND RESCUE

So far in this book I've talked a lot about some serious calls and some grim situations. For readers who are thinking about a career in EMS, or thinking, "Man, I could never do that," it's important to understand that these kinds of calls represent probably only 10 to 15 percent of the job. Most of the time, calls are routine: people who experience shortness of breath or chest pain, or who have fallen and broken a bone. I often tell people who are thinking about a career in EMS, that if they've been a parent and dealt with cuts, scrapes, bumps, bruises, vomiting, and runny noses, if they can do that, then they can do this job, because 90 percent of it is exactly that.

It's about holding somebody's hand, being somebody's friend for twenty minutes. It's about calming people down. For our patients the experience may be personal chaos, but for us, it's very basic diagnostics. It's about putting a monitor on; it's about putting an IV in; it's about putting some oxygen on; and it's about calming patients down to the point where those procedures can do their job. It may involve a medication or two. It might involve none of that, and it may just be that the patient needs a ride to the hospital to be checked out.

There's a housing complex for the elderly in our community. People who live alone, who may not have family visitors, can panic when something doesn't feel right. If their only support is the fire department and the ambulance, they call 9-1-1. It's very common for us to be called in to do a blood pressure check, check their medicine, give them a pat on the shoulder, and tell them they're okay.

This one little old lady, Sylvia, was transported routinely. She was a diabetic. She had a heart condition and anxiety attacks. She started to hyperventilate, and then she felt light headed as though she were going to pass out. Just before that happened, she did one of two things: she either sucked on her inhaler, which raised her heart rate and made her even more light headed so she called 9-1-1, or she just called 9-1-1 and skipped the inhaler part. Her apartment was well known to everybody. She was on a first name basis with almost everyone in the fire department and all of the medics. She was the sweetest little old lady; she was eighty-eight years old, and her apartment was impeccably taken care of.

Little figurines were everywhere, doilies on all the tables; it was exactly what you would expect your grandmother's apartment to look like. When we got there, she was sitting in her chair with her afghan on her lap, and she said, "Oh, hi, boys." She had pictures of her kids and pictures of her grandkids. We'd never met any of them, all the times we'd been there, but we all asked her about them. It was never anything serious, but we were there once a week because it was part of our job.

Calls like Sylvia's are the reset button for us; they help to temper all of the ugliness of the critical calls. There are days when we go without anything serious, days when I put four hundred miles on the truck, going from call to call to call, and all of them turn out to be basic level calls with nothing for me to do.

It's not full speed all the time. It's a people business and it's about caring for people whether they are in personal panic mode but without real distress, or whether they're in a life-threatening situation.

No matter how long you've been in this career, everybody's adrenalin pumps up when the call is for a little kid, whether it's either one of our own who's hurt or someone else's. We will race to wherever the incident is when a kid has been injured.

I remember a little kid, probably five years old, who had belly pain. His parents said he had a fever, and just really wasn't feeling good, and was just all freaked out by the fact that he had to go to the hospital. I got to the scene and I hopped in the back. His mom was there. This kid's eyes were the size of half dollars; he looked at me, and all my equipment, and just started screaming. I don't usually get that response.

I introduced myself to his mom. "I'm Bob. I'm one of the paramedics from the hospital. What's going on?"

"He's had abdominal pain in his lower right side for the last couple of days, and now he can't sit still."

"Got a fever?"

"Yes."

"Okay, and he hasn't been able to sleep?"

"No."

"Can't touch it?"

"Nope."

I laid him flat on stretcher in the ambulance. Mom told me his name was Toby.

The kid said, "You going to give me a needle?" Dead serious.

"I'm going to try not to."

"I don't want any needles. If you're going to give me a needle, I don't like you."

"Okay, Toby, fair enough. How about if I just check your belly and we decide from there what needs to be done? Will you let me do that?"

"Is it going to hurt?"

"It might when I get to the lower part."

One thing I teach all my students is not to lie to patients. If it's going to hurt, tell them it's going to hurt, because if you lie to them, you'll break their trust, especially when it comes to kids, and you'll have no credibility with them from that point forward. If you tell them, "It might hurt a little bit, but I need to figure out what's going on so that I can help you," things go much better.

"Oh...okay."

"All you have to do is just lie flat. I'm going to press down, and then I'm going to let go. I need you to tell me if it hurts, and if it hurts more when I press in, or when I let go. I'm going to do it four times. Okay?"

"Yeah, I can do that."

I was looking for something called rebound tenderness to see if it hurt more when I let go than when I pressed down, because rebound tenderness is typical of appendicitis. When you assess a patient, you always begin where you know it doesn't hurt, and end with where you know it's going to hurt the most. If you immediately start where it hurts, their anxiety level goes up. If you've already touched them two or three times in your assessment before you get to the painful area, they think, "Okay. This isn't so bad." So I started on the upper left side, knowing it wouldn't hurt, and worked my way down to the lower right.

"Hurts a little bit," Toby told me.

"Okay." I finally reach the lower right and press down.

He screams, "You hurt me!"

I said, "You knew it might hurt. Okay, we're done." I turned to the mom. "Pretty sure it's appendicitis. We're going to take him in."

A lot of ambulances carry stuffed animals for patients like Toby, so the EMT pulled out a teddy bear and a dog, and asked, "Which one do you like?"

"The dog."

"Great. Now, Toby, what do you want to name the dog?"

"Rescue."

"All right. We'll call him Rescue."

Toby and Rescue and Mom and I went to the hospital.

I asked Toby, "Do you want the basic ride, or do you want the VIP, super special five-year-old ride?"

"I want that one."

There's an intercom between the front and the back of the truck and I said, "Driver? Toby, would like the VIP ride, please."

"Absolutely, sir,"came the reply.

On went the siren and the lights, which we were going to use anyway.

"This is the very special ride. We're going to use the siren all the way in, just like you see in TV."

"Cool."

"You can tell all your friends you got the VIP ride to the hospital."

It was a nice steady ride, because there was no reason to go fast. By the time we arrived at the hospital, Toby had perked up a little bit.

I asked him, "How was that?"

"That wasn't so bad." And he reached over and asked me, "What's your name again?"

"It's Bob. You remember? You're Toby; that's Rescue; I'm Bob."

"Thanks for not putting a needle in me. That was good."

"I can't promise that's going to continue for the rest of the day, buddy, but for now, we're cool. You and Rescue—I'll check in on you later. You do well, and make sure that Mom gives you ice cream later on, tomorrow."

His eyes lit up. "Really?"

"Yep, with a special ride like this, you'll probably stay overnight. You might even be in for a day or so, but afterward, ask for ice cream. Bet you'll get it."

His mom carried him in, and gave me a grateful look over her shoulder. Toby and Rescue, that's part of what the job is. It's not all chaos. Sometimes, it's about just being a person.

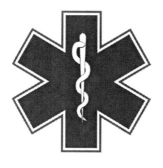

CHAPTER 20

PANCAKES, A POLICE CHASE, AND A HELICOPTER

PANCAKES, A POLICE CHASE, AND A HELICOPTER

When the paramedic program started, we really didn't have a dedicated office where we could go in between calls. We were kind of stuck in the truck, at the hospital in the emergency department, or hanging out at one of the local firehouses where we could slump in a chair and catch a catnap. One of the other places where we used to hang out was the local International House of Pancakes. It was great to go there around midnight and have a late dinner, because we were on duty until seven in the morning. It was fun because the bars would start to empty out and we could watch the festivities. The drunks would come in and try to sober up, and the guys who were trying to get somewhere on their first dates would come in, hoping that they didn't sober up the girls they were with too much.

Every once in a while, we'd wind up breaking up a fight, when a couple of drunks would get into one, and we'd all stand up in uniform and tell them, "You really should stop now," as we got on the radio and asked for a cop. The IHOP people loved having us there, because we were kind of unofficial bouncers. Nobody knew what the heck we were, but we were in uniform, with radios and stuff hanging off our belts, so we had a peace-keeping effect. Every once in a while, the manager would underwrite our check as a thank-you.

One night, four of us were sitting around: Todd, who was working with me; the other medic, Cody and his partner Brian. All of us were having pancakes and coffee. One of the guys had a scanner and we'd been bantering back and forth about which of us was going to do the "bad one" that night. Cody was giving as good as he got: "Don't worry, we've got the serious stuff. You guys are going to be picking up the slack."

Todd and I didn't back down: "Nah, we've got all the serious stuff. You can just take care of grandma and do all the routine calls."

Just as we finished dinner, Cody and Brian were called out to a local convalescent home for a ninety-one-year-old woman with breathing difficulty.

"See?" I said. "You guys take care of the routine stuff. We're going to go call the helicopter."

"Screw you; we'll be back."

As Todd and I walked out to the truck, we heard a police chase on the scanner, coming from the next town and right up the street where the IHOP was. It was going to come right by us.

"Sounds like entertainment; let's go watch," I said to Todd.

We got in the truck. A little Ford Escort and cruisers—one, two, three zipped by. They were heading out toward the interstate as if they were going to get on the highway and head toward New London. We were Medic 11, which was assigned to the New London side of the river, so I said, "Let's follow it. How far can an Escort go before it crashes? We might as well be near the crash scene when it happens."

We followed behind the cruisers as they headed up the ramp, far enough back that we didn't interfere or get in the way. We also looked in our rear-view mirror for other cops so that we could get out of their way too. The ramp went to I-95 southbound. We watched the Escort get to the end of the ramp, and take a right, going *north* in the southbound lanes.

"This is not going to be good," I said to Todd.

The exit ramp dumped southbound traffic into the high-speed lane, and the driver of the Escort had just taken a right turn, so he was now going northbound at high speed in the southbound lanes on a Friday night. One cruiser zipped across the highway and started going north, with his lights on, in the breakdown lane, trying to warn traffic what's coming. The two cruisers stopped in case the Escort driver realized what he'd done and turned around to come back.

No sooner did I get the words "Do you want to follow the cop up the breakdown lane?" out of my mouth when we heard a tremendous crash.

"Let's go. We'll take our chances."

Todd hit our lights and siren, and we went past the other cruisers. One of them got in behind us, and we headed northbound into the breakdown lane. Coming up over the rise, we hadn't gone three hundred yards before we see the Escort, sitting sideways, with a tandem tractor-tailor buried in the passenger side of the car. Clearly, the guy was going up the highway, saw the truck at the last minute, and tried to swerve to the left. But the truck couldn't stop, so it just clobbered the car.

As we pulled in, we saw the first cop that had been chasing the Escort getting out and running over with a fire extinguisher. I could see a little bit of a fire in the engine compartment of the Escort. He turned around and stared at us as if we were from Mars, and asked, "Where the hell did you guys come from?"

"We saw which way he went and we figured you could use us."

Car parts were still ricocheting around the highway, rolling to a stop. We grabbed the fire extinguisher off the medic truck, and

I went running over to the car where the cop was standing, Todd behind me. We could see right away that the Escort driver was critically injured. There was a fire in the engine compartment near him, but, so far, it was far enough away from him not to be an immediate threat.

"All right, you take the extinguishers," I said to the cop. "Todd, I'll start the assessment; you grab a board and collar, but make it quick; we've got to get him the hell out of here."

Todd went back and grabbed the backboard. I started taking care of the guy, holding his head so he couldn't move if he woke up, and I tried to assess his injuries.

I had visions of the two girls call, because the scene looked the same: facial injuries from the flying glass, and the passenger door up against the gear shift. I saw the semi's grill, which was now in what would have been the passenger door window.

The trucker asked what he could do to help, yelling, "I couldn't stop. I couldn't stop." He was obviously upset.

"Go turn your truck off. We don't need any more combustion issues."

He turned off the diesel engine. Now I could at least think without the diesel engine in my ear. Todd came back with the backboard, and we did the fastest rapid extraction we'd ever done. Luckily for us, the stars aligned and he wasn't caught on anything. As we pulled him out, I saw the cop manning the extinguisher. "Do me a favor: just don't squirt me with the extinguisher. Keep the fire back."

But the fire was getting out of control, and the cop was not able to keep up with the extinguisher. He'd used up his, so now he was using ours. We pulled the guy out as far away as we could on the highway and straight up the lane that we were in, because the tractor-trailer was already blocking that lane. Cars were still trying to pass us, because they had no idea why the tractor-trailer had stopped. I was anticipating the next crash, which I figured would happen when someone came screaming around the bend and hit the back of the stopped tractor-trailer.

Once we were away from the burning car, I called the dispatch center on my portable. "Medic 11 to fire alarm, we need the status on Lifestar. Can they launch?" It was cloudy and foggy, so we weren't sure if weather conditions would permit them to launch the helicopter.

Over the hospital's frequencies I heard Cody's voice. "Cut the crap. Be serious."

I keyed the microphone again. "Medic 12, I haven't got time for this. We're for real."

I heard a "Yeah, whatever," as they pulled into the convalescent home to take care of the little old lady. They thought we were messing around with them. They hadn't heard any of the police chase, and they had no idea what had gone on in the six minutes since they had left.

Dispatch came back with, "Lifestar is not available because of weather. You're going to have to do it by ground."

"Okay. No problem. Send the ambulance."

The state and local police responded and blocked the highway off behind us, so there was a wall of cruisers behind the truck. Nothing could get by them, which at least it made the area safe to walk around in without getting clobbered by a passing car.

"Medic 11, tell the ambulance the road's closed. Have them come up the on ramp for southbound, turn north, and come up to the accident scene. It's only three hundred yards up the highway. Then back in and we'll load from there."

The guy was just mangled. There was nothing we could do for him, other than backboard him, put a collar on him, and put IVs in him. He wasn't breathing. I knelt in the middle of the interstate, trying to intubate him but his airway had shifted. That is a sign of several things, all of them bad.

I put a large IV needle into his chest to try and decompress it. This is the fastest way to rule out the cause of the shifted airway. I got a rush of air and a spray of bright red blood from the catheter so I knew that not only did he have pressure caused by a collapsed lung and air trapped in his chest, I also knew he had bleeding in his chest, which I couldn't do anything about. He was also in cardiac arrest, and it was clear that he was not coming back. Even so, we did CPR on him all the way to the hospital.

When we got there, the docs took one look at him. "How long's he been down? What happened?"

"He got clobbered by a semi. He was doing 60 mph plus in an Escort and ran smack into a tractor-trailer. We had a pulse when we started. He hasn't been breathing since we got there. We lost the pulse. I decompressed his chest. We've done three rounds of meds, hung two bags of fluid, and I'm not getting any response. I don't even have a shockable rhythm. Got a flatline, nothing."

The docs said, "Okay. We're done."

That was the end of it.

Afterward, we cleaned up. The ambulance was littered with bandages, intubation tube wrappers, syringes, boxes of medication, IV starter kits, and tape. Blood was everywhere and we hosed it down. We heard the backup alarm for an ambulance coming in beside us. It was the Mystic ambulance that Cody was on, bringing in that ninety-one-year-old with shortness of breath. They had to go the long way to the hospital because the highway was closed. I stood there, dripping wet with sweat. We took a broom and swept out the ambulance because there was so much garbage in it.

Cody looked in and his face fell. "I thought you were kidding."

"I told you. You guys do the routine stuff, and we'll handle the trauma. We couldn't even get the helicopter. We just did it ourselves."

He growled. "Shut the hell up." He took his patient in to get her second breathing treatment. He has never, to this day, let me forget that. "You guys. Pancakes and helicopters, pancakes and helicopters."

We still laugh about it. When I see those guys, I say, "Want to go to IHOP?"

"Shut up."

"Okay."

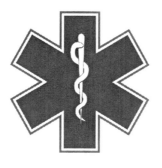

CHAPTER 21

HOT-WIRED

HOT-WIRED

Over the course of my career, there have been three calls involving high voltage electricity. Because of that, I will admit that I won't do any kind of electrical work. I'll change a light bulb, but if it comes to changing out lights or wires, I'm not touching it. I've got a very healthy fear of electricity.

Early on, when I was working in Meriden, in bad winter weather we'd pull out the reserve fleet of Cadillac ambulances because they drove better in the snow. During one such shift Ed and I were responding to a motor vehicle accident reported as a "car versus pole." We started to slow down because we could see the accident up the street a little way and it was dark. We wanted to make sure wires weren't down and we weren't stepping someplace we shouldn't. All we could see was what was in front of our headlights. We crept onto this scene, and I could see the cops were on the other side of the accident. At the last possible second, I saw something, and I yelled at Ed to stop. A wire was hanging across the road at the windshield level of the ambulance. He stopped, but not quickly enough. We hit the wire, and it wrapped itself around the bubble light on the top. The end of it came down and draped itself around the spotlight on my door. I was sitting on the passenger side of the ambulance with my window down, and if the wire had gone another foot, it would literally have come into the window and landed in my lap. The thing arced and the current actually burned a hole in the side of the vehicle. I came within a foot of being electrocuted.

We ended up trapped in the ambulance. When you have a live wire on your vehicle, you stay in it, because if you open the door and put your feet on the ground, you connect the circuit, and you can be electrocuted and die. Ed reached for the radio, and I jerked his hand back. I didn't know any better and thought he might be electrocuted. We ended up using the portable radio to call our dispatch center and tell them we were stuck with a live wire on the ambulance, and that they needed to send another ambulance. "You need to get the power company to come rescue us, because we can't get out of the vehicle."

We were trapped in the ambulance for probably thirty minutes before the power company guy came over and said, "We've shut it off. You can get out."

We were both kind of nervous, and I said, "Do me a favor. Pull the wire off the truck, and then I'll believe you."

"Okay." He grabbed it with his big linesman gloves, and we got out. By that time the other ambulance had come, taken the patient, and left. That was incident number one, and it shook me up.

Several years later, I was working in Hartford after hurricane Gloria came through and had done some pretty significant damage, including causing a lot of power outages. Some circuits were still up, and the power company was trying to leave as many circuits on as possible, which meant there were some live wires in places that people weren't supposed to be, at least according to the power company.

There's a park on the West Hartford line called Elizabeth Park. It's very famous for its rose garden, and it's popular with walkers and for winter sledding, including ambulance crew tobogganing. We were called to Elizabeth Park for a kid who had been electrocuted.

On our arrival we found that the Hartford Fire Department's rescue truck had gotten there ahead of us. The victim, a teenaged kid, was sitting on a log near a tree that had had yellow tape marked "DO NOT CROSS" wrapped around it. The kid was kind of bent over. Steam was coming off him, and yellow tape was wrapped round him too.

The rescue truck guy said to me, "He's out of it, man. He's gone."

"What do you mean, gone?"

"Listen to him. He's making no sense."

I went over to the kid, introduced myself, and said, "Do you know where you are?"

He did.

I said, "Do you know what happened to you?"

"I got zapped," was his answer.

But between answering my questions, he recited the alphabet, going through the alphabet forward and then backward. And I realized what the firefighter meant: this kid was crazy.

We found out from a friend that the kid had walked into a bush to urinate, but there was a live wire in the bush, and he got entangled in it. It wrapped around him, and just kept zapping him. I wanted to cut his clothes off to see how bad the injuries were. He'd been zapped so hard that part of his clothes had actually melted to his body.

Holy crap. Okay. He has third degree burns and his clothing is melted onto him. I have to figure out how to manage him and get him out of here.

We laid him on the stretcher, put him on oxygen, covered him in a sheet to minimize contamination of his burned skin areas—about 50 percent of his body—and screamed to the hospital, which immediately shipped him up to Shriners Burn Hospital in Boston.

When electricity enters your body, especially high voltage electricity, it enters at a point of contact, travels throughout your body, and, typically, exits. That exit point is actually another wound, and based on where the current exits, you can estimate where the current may have gone in the body. If you have an entrance wound in a hand, and an exit wound in a foot, theoretically you can have cardiac problems and all sorts of issues, because the electricity wreaks havoc. It creates a burn; it creates a wound, and it creates havoc with your nerves, muscles, and your cardiac system. You have to look at the whole body to figure out what could be going on.

The boy actually had three exit wounds: an exit wound in one of his buttocks, an exit wound on the bottom of one of his feet, and an entrance and exit wound in his hand, where he came in contact with the wire, thinking it was a branch. That's how it started: he went to move a branch and hit the wire. When it zapped him, he pulled back, and when he did that, the wire came down and zapped him some more, until finally the circuit blew out and stopped. The boy got to Boston, but he ended up losing one of his feet and needing multiple skin grafts because of his third degree burns.

More than a year later I wound up going to court as a witness, and my documentation of the incident served as one of the pieces of evidence used to help win the case for this kid. The fire department's report had said that he was incoherent, and that was translated by the power company's attorney to say that he might have been under the influence of alcohol. My report stated was that he wasn't incoherent; he was mumbling, reciting the alphabet forward and backward, trying to keep himself sane until someone came to take care of him. He knew who he was, where he was, and what had happened to him, and he showed no sign of being under the influence of alcohol.

Outcomewise, he did relatively well. He was a high-school athlete in really, really good shape, and he ended up helping to develop some prosthetic devices for other kids, because he was in such good shape they could use him to test them. But his burned skin and the damage that had been done to him made me realize once again that—holy crap!—electricity was not something I wanted to mess with.

The third call came right after we become paramedics down in New London and, again, the call was for a car versus telephone pole with wires down. I was working with another medic that night, Mike. We responded with the New London Fire Department ambulance. The two firefighter/EMTs on duty that night were guys we worked with all the time. So the four of us were well acquainted.

I had chest pain on the way to this call, because I was in a truck responding to a call in which downed electric cables were involved. The last time I had done this, the downed wire had burned a hole in the vehicle. I had flashbacks to the call in Meriden.

I really, really hate electricity.

We rolled in to find that the car had driven directly through a telephone pole, and taken out the middle section; it looked like a cartoon. The top was hanging by the wires, and the bottom was intact. But there was no driver. The car was there, the damage was there, the wires hung across the street. We stepped out of the truck and saw a guy lying on his lawn.

"Is that the driver?" we asked the cop.

"No, but that's your patient. We don't know where the driver is. There's damage to the car, obviously; you can see the wires and every-thing else. We don't know where he went. We've got guys looking for him. We don't know if he's in the bushes, or if he just ran away. This guy came out to see the accident, saw fire on his lawn in the dark, didn't know what it was, stepped on it, and got electrocuted trying to put the fire out. And when he got electrocuted, he fell on the wire. So the wire's underneath him, and it's still live."

The four of us stood there, helpless. We couldn't touch him, because if we did, we'd be electrocuted. The power company had yet to arrive, and this guy was literally on a live wire. The fire department crew was going to try to roll him off with a long wooden pole called a pike pole and linesman gloves, but they didn't know what the voltage level was, and wood can conduct electricity. If the voltage is very high, it can go right up the pole. The four of us were helpless. We couldn't do a thing.

We'd got the gear ready to go. We knew we were going to have to put the victim on the monitor and probably defibrillate him to try to get him back. We watched this guy lying there smoking. He was cooking. There's no other way to put it.

When we arrived, he was breathing, but now he wasn't and time was ticking. We looked at each other. Everybody saw him stop breathing. We were keeping track of time, so we knew how long we had to save him when we did manage to get to him. We knew we were going to have to deal with the after-effects of an electrocution. We also knew we were going to have to deal with a fairly severe burn to his back, because he was lying on his back on this wire.

The power company guy arrived. We heard the hiss of his air brakes. Just as he pulled in, the weight on the wires finally brought down the remains of the telephone pole. The wires started swinging, and the transformer on the pole came plummeting down into the street and exploded. Sparks showered everywhere. We ducked for cover on the other side of the power company truck, but we didn't know where the wires would go. As we ducked for cover, we saw the guy bounce up off the lawn as if we had hit him with the defibrillator.

"Whoa! Everybody see that?"

All four heads were going up and down. "Yep."

We looked at his chest going up and down.

"He wasn't breathing before, right? You guys all saw that?"

"He wasn't breathing, man. I'm positive. We all saw it. Now he is."

The power company guy ran over. "It's clear. Power's off. You're safe to touch him now."

We went over and put him on the monitor. He had a very slow respiratory rate. We rolled him over and saw this S-shaped, third-degree burn on his back. We put him into the ambulance, rolled him onto his side, and dressed the burn.

Suddenly he woke up and looked up at us. "What happened?"

The guy from the fire department said, "Dude, you are the luckiest guy I have ever met. When you get out of the hospital, you need to go buy lottery tickets."

We went back to the scene afterward to talk to the power guy and pick up some equipment that we had forgotten. The guy told us, "Yes, the transformer blew and sent a shock through the line."

I said, "Listen, if you're going to start defibrillating patients for us, tell us now. We don't need to respond if you're going to do it."

"What are you talking about?"

So we told him the story.

"No shit."

The guy ended up going to the burn center down in Bridgeport. It turned out that he had a cardiac history. All four of us swore that he was absolutely, positively not breathing, and was defibrillated by the power company. All we did was put him on the monitor, put him on oxygen, and take him in. He woke up in the ambulance, went down to Bridgeport—and was released. When he went home, he sold his house and moved. To this day, the four of us still say, "Remember the electrocution call?"

It was insane.

Those three instances have convinced me that when there's electrical work to be done in my house or my office, electricians can do it. I don't. In the words of Clint Eastwood, "A man's got to know his limitations." When it comes to home repair, my limitation is to write the check.

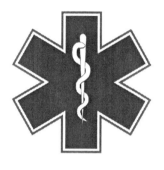

CHAPTER 22

A MARRIAGE AND FOUR SUICIDES

A MARRIAGE AND FOUR SUICIDES

By 1993 my life was still crazy busy but working for me. I was running my consulting business and working in New London on the medic truck—and I'd met a nurse and fallen in love with her. Debbie and I got married.

It seemed like a great idea at the time. Debbie and I had a great first six or seven months together, and then the differences between us—we were both strong-willed, stubborn people—overwhelmed the good. I had no need to be taken care of, and Deb had a strong desire to care for someone. Nurses tend to be very good caregivers, but I saw myself as a caregiver, too, not a needy person. The head-butting between us commenced very shortly after we got married, and we spent another eighteen months in limbo together, both of us separately contemplating whether we wanted to split or to stay together, going to work, coming home, going through the motions. It finally got to the point that we'd each cringe when we'd hear the garage door open and we'd know the other person was coming home. I fell back on my old habits and threw myself more into work to stay out of the house.

It was the week between Christmas and New Year's Day in '95 when Debbie finally asked me, "Do you want a divorce?" and I said, "Yes." We were separated the following week, even though we ended up living together for probably another three or four months while we sorted things out financially. I spent that three months living on the couch, going to work, and staying out. Fortunately, the demands of a start-up business and my medic truck shifts were more than enough to keep me busy.

During this period I was dispatched to a call in one of the fairly rural towns in the service area for a possible gunshot wound. The weather was horrendous; wind-swept rain came down in buckets. The road was flooding, which made our response time slower. We couldn't see more than a few feet ahead of us through the torrential downpour.

I turned to my partner, Jeff, at one point during the response, and asked, "How can there be a gunshot wound in this kind of weather? Who's stupid enough to be out in this?"

We got to the scene, an old farmhouse, and pulled in the driveway, where there was one cruiser. The cop was standing out in the driveway in his DayGlo, lime-green raincoat. I got out of the truck and said, "Is this real? Do we really have a shooting?"

"Well, yeah, but you're not going to have to do much."

Okay, there had to be more to this story.

"Where is he? In the house, in the garage, where?"

"No, he's in the woods."

"He's where?"

"He's in the woods. He's over there."

Over in the doorway of the house, I saw a young lady, probably in her mid-twenties, obviously distraught, crying, and holding her hands over her mouth as if she couldn't believe what was going on.

"Who's that?"

"That's the daughter."

"Okay. Where's our victim?"

"Go down the path between the garage and the house, all the way back to the clearing in the woods."

"Do I need anything?"

"Just whatever you need to do a presumption."

"Okay. You called me all the way out here in this for that?"

"Sorry, I've got to. It's protocol."

"Okay."

We grabbed the monitor, and I took everything just in case, because sometimes people could be wrong, especially if they had done a quick assessment. I didn't know this particular officer, so I didn't know his skill level. We followed the path into the woods, going back probably fifty to seventy-five feet on this fairly well-worn path, and we reached a clearing. Water was pouring off me in sheets. I was concerned that if we had to actually use the defibrillator for any reason, we were going to kill ourselves. How was I going to defibrillate anybody in this kind of weather? I was also afraid that the monitor was going to be damaged by all the rain. Still, I had to take it.

Entering the clearing, I literally couldn't believe what I was looking at. A gentleman was sitting in a plastic lawn chair up against a tree. On the ground was a travel coffee mug, and a hunting rifle had fallen into his lap. The coffee mug was sitting in what was clearly a well-worn spot, where he'd always set it down, and the chair was in a spot that was obviously a favorite. If you looked from where he was sitting, you could see up the path to his house, and his garage, and you had a view of his property. This was plainly a special place for him. But this was also what he had decided would be a good place to end his life. He had taken a hunting rifle, put it in his mouth, and pulled the trigger. There was nothing for us to do.

Even in the rain I could tell that this had happened a while ago. The blood had congealed, and there was brain matter on the tree. The conditions met every bit of our protocol to presume the man dead right there and not transport him but turn him over to the medical examiner and leave. But we had to go through the exercise just to make sure.

So, I reached over and checked a pulse and put the stethoscope on his chest and auscultated for a heartbeat. That was the protocol. There was enough trauma to his head for me to know that I didn't need to put the actual monitor on him, but we had to go through the procedure. It was about two in the afternoon, so we officially presumed him at 2:01 pm.

We went back to the house to talk to his daughter. We found out her father was seventy-seven years old. I asked her, "Why there? Why today? Was he upset about something?"

She said, "My mom died ten years ago, and he hasn't really been right since. That was his favorite spot. The two of them used to sit out there together. He used to go back there all the time and just sit there with a cup of coffee."

She told us that they used to have a bench back there that they'd shared. It had become overgrown over the years because he hadn't taken care of it, but it was still the spot he associated with his wife. He had been diagnosed with cancer and had beaten it, but the week before this had happened, his doctor had told him that the cancer had come back. He just could not face another round of chemo and another round of treatment, and decided that seventy-seven was a good age to go. He'd decided he was ready to be with his wife, so this morning, along with his coffee, he'd taken his hunting rifle.

I said, "Is there anything we can do for you?"

She said, "No. It was a shock to find him, and it was a shock that he did it, but it wasn't all that surprising. He's been talking a lot about my mother in the last week. I knew he wasn't going to be comfortable going through it again, so this was his way of taking himself out the way he wanted to go."

We put everything back in the truck, gave her phone numbers for mental health or counseling if she needed it, and gave the cop our information. You have to give the police officer your name, badge number, and time of death, so he has that information for his report. We got back into the truck and left. We decided we were going to go down the street and get a cup of coffee, and we pulled into the coffee shop.

"Man, I can't believe how wet it is out here," I said. "I am literally just soaked." As I was talking, I reached into my wallet to pull out some money to pay for the coffee, and water ran out of my wallet. It had rained so much down into the back pockets of my pants that literally everything I had was soaked.

"We should get coffee and go change."

"Yeah, that'd be good," Jeff said.

That experience made me look harder at my own life. I thought about what was going through that guy's mind that he could have such a strong relationship with somebody he was willing to die to be back with her. I thought about my own situation and wondered if I'd ever have that depth of feeling for anybody. The notion that someone could get so despondent he'd take his own life seemed so strange to me.

About a month later, I got another call for a gunshot wound. When we arrived, we found a couple of cops standing at the door, and the first thing one of them said to me was, "I don't think there's much you can do for this guy."

Hmm, I'm seeing a recurring pattern here.

Different town this time, but same situation. The other cop shook his head. He had this smirk on his face.

"What could possibly be funny about this?" I asked him.

"I'll tell you the story later. Go do what you've got to do and come back, and I'll tell you the story. I'm still having trouble buying off on this one, but it's a funny story."

"Okay."

Sick bastard.

The house was fairly new. There were still stickers on a couple of windows, and I could smell fresh paint, except in the room where the victim was, the master bedroom. This guy had lain across the bed, propped himself up with pillows against the headboard, stuck a shotgun in his mouth, and blown the top of his head off.

The inside of the house looked like a Charles Manson crime scene, because blood was everywhere, spattered all over the wall, all over the bed, all over the carpet, everywhere. It was obvious there was absolutely nothing that we could do there except to presume him dead. Because I had to, I auscultated the man's heart. Sometimes, even though there's that much damage to the brain, the mechanical portion of the heart doesn't know enough to stop. This shooting seemed to have happened a very short time earlier. I confirmed there was no heartbeat. We presumed him dead at 4:37 pm.

I went out to talk to the cop. "Who found him?"

"She found him." The cop pointed to a very distraught woman sitting in the living room.

"His wife?"

"No. His exwife. She comes home from work at about four thirty, so he waited for her."

"Well, at least he did it to himself and didn't take her out."

"Oh, no. The story is even more interesting than that," the cop said.

"Okay."

"The exwife is remarried. This is *their* new house."

It was quite a story. The dead exhusband had never gotten over the fact that his wife had broken up with him. The anger just kept building and building and building. It didn't help that he was hearing from all of their exfriends that "she's doing really well, so happy, so successful." One day he lost his job, and that was the last straw for him. He had lost his job. He had lost his wife. She was doing really well. She had remarried. She had a new house.

He lost it.

He broke into his exwife's new home, broke into her bedroom, set himself on her bed, put a shotgun in his mouth, blew his head off all over their wall, and left a note on her dresser, which read, "I hope you two are happy together."

"This is funny to you?" I asked the cop.

"It's just my sick sense of humor. What do you want from me? It just struck me as strange that the guy would go to all this trouble to break into his ex's house and off himself."

I just stared at him. He shrugged and looked away. "I was thinking about *my* ex."

Ah, okay.

"You've got a sick mind."

He glanced at me again and shrugged. "Well, yeah, whatever."

A couple of weeks later we were driving by the scene on the way to another call and saw a "For Sale" sign on the house.

In an unexpected way, those two relationship-related calls put some stuff in perspective for me, made me think about where I was in my own relationship, as opposed to where I thought I'd be in my life. I knew there had to be more.

As I thought about it all, another call from years before came to mind too. It's a funny thing that I've noticed through my career: I might forget altogether about a particular call from years back until something, a scent, a sound, happens to bring it all rushing back from the depths of memory.

This particular call was in a very, very wealthy neighborhood in a suburb of Hartford. We'd been called to a possible overdose. We got there and found a seventeen-year-old girl—absolutely gorgeous, long blonde hair, the quintessential cheerleader look, which in fact she was. She was a smart girl, I found out afterward from her parents, who were both distraught. Some things had happened recently in the girl's life that she just couldn't deal with. Dad would not leave his daughter's side. Mom was in the other room sobbing. It had been hours from the time the daughter had gotten home from school to the time the parents had returned home, found her, and called us.

She was lying in bed. She was cyanotic, which gives the skin a bluish tinge. She was cold. We were way past the time to be able to do anything; she'd been dead for quite a while. A bottle of Mom's sleeping pills sat by the side of the bed. It was empty. I looked at it and saw that the prescription had been refilled approximately a week before. I asked the mother, "Just for the record, how many of these did you use?"

She said, "There were fifty tablets in the bottle. I probably used five."

So the girl had washed down forty-five sleeping pills with some alcohol, and they had depressed her respiratory system to the point where she just died in her sleep. But what would drive this absolutely stunningly beautiful, intelligent seventeen-year-old girl to do this?

In talking to her mom, I learned that her daughter had been recently diagnosed as a type 1 diabetic. She did not want to deal with the disease and having to take daily Insulin shots. She had passed out at school a couple of times because she wasn't able to regulate her sugar levels. Kids had made fun of her, and her boyfriend had decided that he didn't want to be associated with her disease either, because it wasn't a cool thing. He had dumped her, and had told her he'd dumped her because there was something wrong with her. The father had been trying to setup some counseling to help her deal with her illness, because these kinds of issues are very common with young kids that have early onset diabetes.

When kids have to travel with insulin and syringes, it's tough. Often they don't take care of themselves because they still feel they're invincible; they don't believe the doctors, and they stay in denial about their disease, so they tend to have lots of episodes of irregular sugar levels. It's not uncommon for them to pass out while they're trying to get used to handling their disease, and other kids can be cruel. Apparently in this particular community, if you weren't perfect, you weren't good enough. She just couldn't handle it; she didn't want to deal with it and decided this was her way out.

She had left a note that said a lot of things: "I love you, Mom and Dad." But the four words that her father could not get out of his head, and probably to this day hasn't been able to get out of his head, were "my life is over," because the boyfriend had dumped her and because she had this disease. Sadly, the way she had decided to cope with her problem made her words come true.

As we drove away, I thought about my own teen years. At seventeen, I was working hard in a restaurant and I had friends. If somebody had said to me, "You're not perfect," or "You're not normal," or "There's something wrong with you," I probably would have said, "Yeah, you're right," and moved on. I just couldn't understand the depth of hurt this girl had felt. This call triggered yet another memory about a call that I had responded to in Hartford probably seven or eight years before, which involved a fourteen-year-old kid.

This kid had come home from school one day, and, again, the parents weren't home. He went into his bedroom, made a noose, put it around his neck, and went down to the basement. There he threw the rope over a beam, climbed on a chair, kicked it away, and hung himself. His mother had been home for three hours before she realized that he wasn't in his room doing his homework. My parents were always there for me, and now that I'm a parent, I try to be there for my kids. I can't imagine being in the house for three hours and not having had contact with my kids, even if it's just to check in and say, "Hey, I'm here. How was your day?" Mom finally went downstairs to do laundry and found her son hanging there.

Again, it was immediately clear that we couldn't do anything for the kid by the time we got there. It was now officially a crime scene. We had to wait for the cops to arrive—which was only another minute or two—so that they could take some photographs before we cut the rope, took the body down, and laid him on the floor.

We ended up having to transport the mother to the hospital, because she was so distraught that her blood pressure was 180/110, which is not good for anybody, but especially not somebody who has other medical problems, as she did, and whose anxiety levels were shooting through the ceiling.

We found out later, from the cop who responded to the call, that this whole incident was over a bad report card and a comment from a teacher. This was the kid's second bad report card in a row, and the teacher had made some comment such as, "You're never going to amount to much the way you're going." It was meant to spur him into action, and it did. The only reason we knew about the report card was that he had taken it down to the basement with him. The mother was furious, determined to go to the school and confront the teacher.

When I ran all these calls together, the common thread that struck me was that the depth of the emotions running through these people's minds was extremely strong. I looked back at all of these cases and thought, *I feel so emotionally disconnected from my life and these people have such powerful emotions that something relatively simple sent them over the edge. I'm on the other side of it. It's almost as if I'm coated in Teflon. My emotions just aren't there.*

It was kind of a freaky realization for me that these people had such strong feelings they could self-destruct over things I'd have dismissed as unimportant.

I was going through a divorce, and I was stuck emotionally on autopilot. Every day I went to work, responded to calls, hung out with my friends, but I was really not as connected to life as I thought I should be. I realized for perhaps the first time that there could be more, and that I needed to find the missing pieces in my own life.

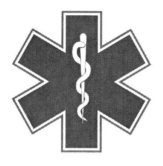

CHAPTER 23

BEGINNINGS AND ENDINGS

BEGINNINGS AND ENDINGS

As usual, I dismissed the thoughts in my head and focused on the present. My consulting business was doing well that year, and it was about then that a woman named Jennifer joined the firm, on July 5, 1994, to be exact. She was hired by one of our managers. I hadn't met her until the day she showed up in the office. We were a small group, just six of us at the time, and we knew each other pretty well. I was married, but it was not going well at all. Jen was engaged, and I learned about four months later that she was not doing well with her engagement. My marriage and her engagement both dissolved on their own; there was nothing between us other than work.

But in 1995 I was separated and getting divorced, and Jen was unengaged. We were invited to a client's holiday party, and we decided to go together. We had a really good time at the party, and I realized that although we knew each other in the work context, we didn't know each other socially.

Hmm. She was a very smart businessperson and a gorgeous woman. We were both officially single. What was I waiting for? I told my sister, Sue, who was also working at the company at the time, "I'm asking Jen out, and if she says yes, she'll be your new sister-in-law."

My sister's smart-assed comment was, "Whoa, big boy. See if you can get her to go out to dinner first."

I'm just telling you.

So I asked Jen if she'd like to have dinner, and to my pleasant surprise she said, "Yeah, I would."

The first time we actually went out was in January '96, and on Christmas Eve '96 we got engaged. The first person I called after Jen said yes to my proposal was my sister. "Your new sister-in-law said yes," I told her.

Jen has always had a love of Christmas, and it was interesting for me because once we started going out and I started to really connect with her, a lot of things changed for me. Normally I would work New Year's Eve. The first year we were engaged was the first year I didn't work that shift, and I have never worked it since. I didn't want to spend as much time at the office. I didn't want to spend as much time on the medic unit. I was finding more reasons not to take a shift than to take one.

In December 1997 we were married. We rented an inn up in Vermont, had fifty of our closest friends and family come for the whole weekend, and everybody hung out together and had a really good time. Christmas has always been a very special time for Jen and me.

After the honeymoon I found myself right back at it, working a lot. Jen understood and was supportive of what I was doing because she was working in the business too. When I did travel, because I was doing consulting projects all over the country, I was gone for a week at a time. It was just the two of us, so it was okay…I thought. I know now that it wasn't.

Five years into our marriage, our kids came along. Parenthood was something I'd originally fought her about. I'd never had kids listed on my master plan…but she did. Thus, in 2001 we officially became pregnant, and as usual, Jen apparently had a buy-one-get-one-free coupon because, in July 2002, twin boys arrived. I have thanked her since that day for the two best gifts I never knew I wanted.

And, full disclosure here, if I knew then what I know now, I'd have embraced the idea from the get-go. I love being a dad.

So, now I had a growing business. I had twin boys. I was still working a shift on the medic unit every Friday, still doing some traveling, and we were trying to manage twin babies. Actually it was Jen who was trying to manage twin babies, and she needed a break.

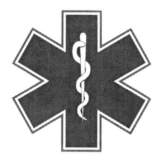

CHAPTER 24

TIME OFF...WELL, NOT REALLY

TIME OFF...WELL, NOT REALLY

Jen and I finally decided that we could manage to take a couple of days to reconnect. The kids were about a year old, so we made plans to go to Florida for the weekend and have some Mom and Dad time. The boys were going to go stay with their aunt. We were leaving on Thursday afternoon and we'd come back on Sunday. We were going to get a couple of days of R&R and some sunshine, and the twins' aunt was going to have a great time taking care of them and doing all kinds of crazy stuff with them. This was the first time Mom had been away from the boys for longer than a few hours, so she was a little conflicted, but we finally separated her from the kids, got on the plane, and settled back.

We sat mid-cabin, right back beside the galley in a big 757 with nice, comfortable seats. We had two seats together, and we held hands. All of a sudden the flight attendant came back, and I saw that she had a worried look on her face. I said to Jen, "This is not going to be good." She rolled her eyes at me as the flight attendant picked up the intercom and made an announcement.

"Attention, ladies and gentleman, is there a doctor aboard? If so, please ring your call button." I put my hand up as she hung up the phone, "I'm not a doctor. Would a paramedic do?"

"Oh, yes. Come with me. We have a sick man up in the front of the cabin."

"Okay. Honey, I'll be back."

Jen just shook her head. "Unbelievable."

I followed the flight attendant up front where this very large man, probably close to 400 pounds, sat with his wife and a couple kids. He looked just horrible. He was sweating bullets.

There's a color that the skin often turns during a heart attack. We call it cardiac grey. I've often joked that it actually ought to be a Sherwin Williams paint color, because everybody in EMS knows it. I look at this guy, and he is cardiac grey.

Oh, no. We're at 30,000 feet.

I asked the flight attendant, "Can you find out where we are? What are we over?"

"We're south of New York and New Jersey."

"What do we have for equipment on board?"

She had oxygen and she had a stethoscope, gloves, and a defibrillator.

I was relieved

"Cool. More than I thought we were going to have."

While I was assessing the man, this other gentleman walked up. "I'm a doctor."

"Excellent. I'm a medic. You want to take over?"

"Mm-mm, not me. I'm a pediatrician. He's bigger than my average patient. I'll help *you*."

The gentleman happened to be a physician from the children's hospital in Hartford.

"Well, can you do me a favor? Talk to the wife and get medications for me while I finish assessing him?"

I put the monitor leads on his chest. It was a defibrillator that had a screen, so I could get a single tracing of the heart rhythm.

When we're in the ambulance we have what's called a 12-lead ECG. We can look at the heart from different points of view to be able to tell what part of the heart is having a problem, so we know what types of symptoms to expect from the patient. For example, if the issue is in the left ventricle, which is the most muscular portion of the heart and the part that pumps the blood to the majority of the body, the patient is likely to go into shock faster and it's likely to be a more severe heart attack.

On the other hand, if the problem is on the right side of the heart, the low-pressure side of the heart that pumps blood to the lungs, it usually takes longer to diagnose, because it masks itself quite often as indigestion or just an uncomfortable feeling. These can sometimes be severe, because they take longer to diagnose.

The monitor that I had to work with only gave me one view of the heart, and it showed an irregular heartbeat.

I put the patient on oxygen and took his blood pressure. He weighed four hundred pounds, and his blood pressure was 90/60. His skin was cool and clammy, so I laid him back in the seat as best I could. There were some empty seats in first class. The flight crew moved his family up there so we'd have more room to work. The first officer came back and asked, "Are we going to be able to continue the flight?"

We were going to Florida. It was a three-hour flight and we were only forty-five minutes into it.

"I don't think so. I have no meds. I can't diagnose him any further. He's got an irregular heartbeat, and he's a big guy with a blood pressure that wouldn't be great for my wife, who's all of 110 pounds. We really need to put this thing down, and have a medic ambulance at the gate to meet us. What's the closest place we can put it down?"

He said, "Best I can do is put it down in DC, which is going to take us another fifteen or twenty minutes to get to."

"That's fine. Pick an airport, put it down, and we'll do what we can."

Once we laid him down, he started to get a little bit better. He still had a little bit of an irregular heartbeat, but he was getting better. So, now I was not really sure whether he'd had an anxiety attack, whether he'd been hyperventilating, or whether he was actually having a cardiac problem; I had no other way of diagnosing it.

After a couple of minutes, his blood pressure improved; it was up to 110/60. His heart rate had slowed down and was a little less irregular. His color was a slightly better with the oxygen. He talked to us a little bit more coherently and comfortably. "I felt like I was going to pass out," he told me. The doctor returned and said the patient was taking two medications, a betablocker, and digoxin, which told me that he had an underlying cardiac problem. With that information I now knew that his heartbeat was probably always irregular. Good. That meant that what I saw on the monitor was probably not new and probably not life-threatening, and it was getting better with the oxygen.

The patient decided he wanted to sit up. I said, "Not a good idea. I'd really rather you stayed like this until we get in."

He said, "No, I really want to sit up." He weighed four hundred pounds and I didn't, so I couldn't argue with him, and I didn't want to stress him out anymore.

"Well, I tell you what. We'll sit you up a little bit. But if you start to have symptoms again, we're going to do it my way."

"All right. That's fair."

The flight crew went through the landing procedure. They told us we'd be landing in about five minutes and that a medic ambulance was standing by. We ended up landing at Reagan National Airport in DC. I told my patient, "Once we get to the gate, the fire guys are at the end of the jetway, waiting."

By the time we landed, he was feeling better. His color had improved. His heart rhythm had probably returned to whatever normal was for him. At that point his blood pressure was 120/70.

The guys from the DC Fire Department came on board and I gave them a full report. They had this little, narrow, chair contraption that was designed for use in the airplane aisle. It was all of fifteen inches wide. I shook my head and smiled at the firefighter holding it.

"What are you going to do with that? He's four hundred pounds."

He just shrugged his shoulders. "It is what it is, man. We'll put another strap on it."

"Okay."

That's just going to give our patient a wedgie.

The patient looked at me. "I don't want to go the hospital. I feel better now, thank you. I don't know what that was. But I feel better, and I really don't want to go."

The fire captain told him, "Well, you don't have to go to the hospital. But once they do an emergency landing, you've got to get off the plane. You just cost the airline a ton of money. So, if you want to sign a refusal of treatment form when you get off the plane, that's fine. But you and your family have got to get off the aircraft."

The guy started to protest. "But we're going on a cruise. We're all going down to Florida." He had just retired a week before. He was going on a cruise with his family.

"I'm sorry," I said to him. "At the time we started this I didn't think you were going to make it all the down way to Florida."

"No, I understand. I understand. It's just kind of a bummer, because the cruise is leaving tomorrow morning."

"I am sure that here is a flight from Reagan down to Florida. The cruise doesn't leave till five. I've been on a lot of them."

As the fire department took him off, the passengers started applauding.

That's a first—the uh-oh squad applauding.

The doc and I shook hands.

"That was a nice job," I said. "Thanks for your help." And I meant it; he was terrific. He'd gotten all the information and even calmed the kids down, which was great, because a pediatrician's used to talking to upset kids. He did a great job with the family so that I could take care of Dad.

Now we were going to wait a while before heading off for Florida, so I sat down.

Jen said, "Really?" She smiled.

"I didn't start it. They called me."

"We can't go anywhere without you running into somebody you know or running into something you've got to help with."

"That's the way it goes, honey."

The flight attendant came over and asked, "Would you like a drink?"

Yes. Yes, we would.

So, we waited on the ground for about an hour, and then took off, went to Florida and had a nice uneventful weekend until Sunday. Coming back we ended up running into really bad weather. It took us an extra day to get home. All the way back Jen was distraught, wanting to get home to the kids.

"That's it. We're not going away anymore. From now on we're taking the kids with us."

"Yes, honey."

The respite was short lived after that trip as we got back into the weekly grind, running the company all week, some travel, and working noon to midnight on Fridays, often coming home at three or four in the morning because of late calls, and then having to get up at six to feed the kids.

Jen said, "Listen, something's got to go. I can't do this by myself."

I realized that there was more to life than running around trying to save everybody else. My family *had* to come first. I realized it. I just didn't do anything about it right away.

Even with all of these blessings, and as happy as things should have been, I was still not easy to live with. I still had all of my emotional baggage. Over the years, I've nearly blown up our marriage on three separate occasions. But we've gotten through it. She stuck by me.

Jen's my best friend. She has taught me what it means to re-engage, to find an emotional spot and to connect with it, and I have to give her credit for saving me, even though I tried my damnedest to screw it up.

As I write this, our sons are now ten, and one is in a cast—stupid bike tricks. I'm probably overly cautious with them because I know what can happen in the blink of an eye. They are probably sick of hearing, "Be careful. Don't do that," but I can't help myself. I've seen too much and know what's out there trying to hurt them. Even so, I can honestly say that parenting is probably the best job I've ever had.

During the last couple years of my career, before Jen convinced me to resign, I still worked noon to midnight every Friday and occasionally a complete overnight shift if they were really jammed up for staff.

One call struck me, just as the suicide calls had struck me, because of the intense emotional connections involved.

It's very common between five thirty and seven thirty in the morning to get calls for people who don't wake up. The dispatch can be anything from "respond to a possible heart attack," or "a person not breathing," or "a possible code," which is our word for cardiac arrest. Some dispatchers actually use the term "untimely," which has always struck me as a funny term for death: an untimely. Nobody really plans on passing away. I guess the guys who commit suicide know when they're going. The rest of us don't have an expiration date on our birth certificates, so any death would be untimely. It was about six fifteen in the morning. I was supposed to get off at seven. I was working alone, covering for a medic who was going to come in a little later.

The call came in for an untimely, and I headed to a neighborhood in an older part of town with a large elderly population. Lots of folks bought their houses in the '40s and the '50s when that neighborhood was built, and they'd lived there all their lives. They'd never moved. The kids grew up in these small, one-story, starter homes in small streets, all with cul-de-sacs and well-kept lawns. When I arrived, I saw an elderly gentleman talking to a police officer I knew well. I could see that the man was teary eyed. I said hello to the cop and asked him, "Billy, where am I going?"

He said, "She's in the kitchen. Go down the hall, last door on the right."

"Okay."

I walked into the kitchen. A woman was lying on the kitchen floor in a flowered, well-worn nightgown. She was in her late seventies, early eighties. She had obviously been there for a while, because she was blue and cold. Just one look and I knew there was not going to be much that we could do. A check proved my suspicions were true. In EMS, we look for signs such as lividity, which is the pooling of blood. When the heart stops, the blood pools in the body, based on the position the body is in. In this case the woman was lying on her back, so the blood had pooled to the back and her skin was dark purple and mottled.

After a short period of time rigor mortis starts to set in. The body becomes very stiff and rigid. That was just starting to happen, so I knew she'd been there for an hour or a little bit longer. The ambulance crew arrived and started to set up their equipment. I looked at them. Surely they could see as well as I could that she was past reviving, but they said, "Listen, we're just going to do this." They had a defibrillator. They put the leads on her chest, and began to load her up. I made eye contact with one of the firefighters I'd known for years and started to say that there was no way we could save her. But before I could say anything, he said, "Go with me on this."

What could I say?

"Okay."

Obviously there was more to the story. They put her on the stretcher, and started taking her out to the ambulance.

I said, "I'll meet you out there."

I was really confused at this point, because normally we would presume this person and we would leave. These guys knew this, yet they were going to take her out in the ambulance and they were going to make it look as if she had a chance.

I went back to talk to the woman's husband, and he just sat there, shaking his head.

"Sir, what's going on?"

He said, "I woke up, and she wasn't there. She's always there. She gets up before me every morning and she goes and gets me coffee, and she comes back, she brings me coffee, and we talk. There was no coffee, and she wasn't there."

He was crying, so I said, "Well, we're going to do whatever we can, and we'll see you at the hospital."

"You going to drive him?" I asked the cop.

"Yeah, I'll bring him down."

I make eye contact with the cop. He knew and I knew and the firemen knew that there was nothing to be done, but there was obviously something going on there. He just nodded his head knowingly. "I'll take care of him."

I went out to the ambulance, got in the back, and closed the doors, and they started to drive away. I put the monitor on, just because I was there. Finally I could ask, "Guys, what are you doing?"

"Listen. It's the mom and dad of one of our department lieutenants, and he just asked that we not leave Mom on the kitchen floor, that we take her to the hospital."

Ah.

"Oh, okay. We're good."

So, I presumed her as we drove. It was a four-minute trip to the hospital. When we arrived at the ER, I said to the doc standing there, "There's no chance. We're not even doing anything. This is for the family's benefit. Just make my presumption official now that we've arrived, so we can say that she died here rather than in the ambulance. The cops are bringing in the husband. If you don't mind, I'll go talk to him and tell him."

"Have at it, man. If I don't have to go make a notification to the family, that's okay with me."

The cop arrived and brought the husband into the emergency department's family room. I went in and asked, "How you doing?"

He reached over, grabbed my hand, and said, "She didn't make it, did she?"

"No, no, she didn't," I said. "We did what we could."

240

"I know. We've been married for sixty years. What do I do? What do I do *now*?"

I said, "I'll be right back." I went to the nurse's station, grabbed a couple of cups of coffee, came back in, and sat next to him. I handed him a cup, and said, "Why don't we start with this?"

He just looked at me with a weak smile and tear-filled eyes. "Thanks."

Shortly after, their son, the lieutenant from the fire department, came in. I knew him pretty well. He walked up to me and said, "I'm glad it was you. Not a chance?"

"No. She must have gotten up at the normal time, and she didn't suffer. There was no trauma or anything. I think she just had had a heart attack, laid down on the floor, and that was it. Your dad didn't wake up, because she didn't come back in. So he got up about an hour later. There really wasn't anything we could do, but we honored your wishes. The guys took good care of your dad. I didn't know the back story, so we took her to the hospital and made it look good for him."

He gave me a hug. "Thanks. I appreciate it."

"No problem. Your dad's in there. He's got his coffee."

"I'll take it from here, man."

It's stuff like that makes this job meaningful, even when it's not full-on chaos. It's some simple act of humanity that you can do to change an outcome for that husband and for the son. We were able to save the husband from having to visualize, every day, his wife dead on the floor. This way, he believed she'd become sick in their house, but she went to the hospital. I wouldn't have known any different. I would have done what I normally do if it hadn't have been for the guys in the fire department. But that's part of the family atmosphere of EMS, fire, and police. It doesn't make a difference to us how we do it, but it matters to those who call on our services.

The part of that story that has always stuck with me was the look on the old man's face when he reached out and asked me, "What do I do *now?*" And after more than two decades of doing this job, I don't have a good answer.

Am I going to be together with my wife for sixty years? I hope so.

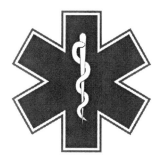

CHAPTER 25

"SEMPER PARATUS": THE U.S. COAST GUARD

"SEMPER PARATUS": THE U. S. COAST GUARD

The cool part about the southeastern Connecticut service area around New London is that it ranges from rural New England farms on one end of the district to typical suburban communities, to an urban environment in the City of New London. When you add to that all of the tourist issues with beaches, an active harbor, nuclear power plants, an active Navy base, and a very, very active waterfront, you have widely varying calls. On one shift, I treated someone who'd fallen off a horse and was stomped. The next call was a shooting in a housing project. It was a fascinatingly diverse area in which to work. In addition, we had not only the U. S. Coast Guard Academy in New London, but also an active Coast Guard rescue station.

It was a Friday afternoon, about twelve thirty. I had literally just come on duty and checked the truck—all the drug boxes, the monitors, and everything else. I closed it up and was going to head out for a cup of coffee. I knew that I was the only medic available, because Medics 11 and 12 were already on calls.

On this particular day I was working by myself. I didn't have a driver with me. The tones went off: "Medic 14 to the Coast Guard station. A sick person on an inbound ferry."

I responded to the Coast Guard station and was met by a petty officer at the gate. He asked, "Anybody with you?"

"Nope, just me. What do you need?"

He pointed to a young uniformed guy next to him. "This is Seaman Adams. He'll help you carry your stuff."

"Okay."

I grabbed the monitor, airway bag, and oxygen. "Where are we going?"

"We've got a 41-footer at the dock for you. You're going to meet the ferry out by the lighthouse."

This was already getting interesting. I went down the stainless-steel gangway, boarded the board, and was handed a life jacket.

I asked, "What's going on?"

The petty officer said, "All I know is that somebody fell down a flight of stairs. They've got a head injury, and they're asking for help. It's going to be easier if we take you to the ferry than if we try to get the person off the ferry and bring him back in, because they're almost at the mouth of the harbor, or they will be by the time we get there."

"Okay."

So, off we went. This was just really cool for me. I was used to being a land-based medic. For some medics, working on boats was routine, not for us.

The blue light's going, siren wailing, and we're racing up to the mouth of the harbor. I was having a good time.

I'm doing a call with the Coast Guard. This is awesome!

We saw the ferry coming in. It was one of the bigger ferries.

As a matter of fact, one of the ferries in New London is actually a converted tank-landing ship that was part of the Normandy invasion on D-Day.

Maybe it will be this one. This will be cool. I'm going to board a ship that was at Normandy.

It turned out to be its sister ship, which had a lower profile in the water.

A crewman told me, "Okay, how this is going to work is that they're going to stop. We're going to pull up alongside the vessel at the stern; it's lower at the car deck, and we're going to pass you and your gear over. Then we're going to escort you back in."

"Okay. Sounds like a plan to me. You guys have done this before. Anything I need to know?"

"Yeah, don't try to jump when the boats are going in opposite directions."

Good advice.

I said, "Do me a favor."

"What?"

"Don't drop the monitor. It costs $15,000 and it doesn't go well with salt water."

"Got it. We're good."

We got there. They brought our vessel alongside. I climbed up over the railing. They handed my gear up to me. "Okay. We'll see you at the dock." They pushed off and headed toward the bow of the ferry to take up the escort duty.

One of the officers from the ferry said, "I'll show you where he is. He fell down a flight of stairs coming from the upper deck, and he's on the mid-deck."

I grabbed my gear, followed him, and soon saw a woman kneeling over the victim, who had a fairly impressive-looking head wound. There was a good-size pool of blood on the deck. We had the uh-oh squad rubbernecking as usual. People were lining the upper deck railing, looking down at this guy. I now had an audience.

I said to the woman, "Are you family? Who are you?"

"No, I'm a nurse. I saw him. He had a seizure on the stairs and fell."

Well, that complicated things. The potential existed for this person, who already had a head injury, to have a seizure. I also didn't know if he'd sustained spinal damage from the fall.

"Did you see him fall?"

"Yeah, he kind of bounced down the stairs, bounced off the railings."

"So, did he fall hard enough that I have a neck injury to deal with?"

"No, I don't think so."

That was hopeful, because I didn't have a backboard or collar with me and there wasn't anything like that onboard.

I said, "Okay. Do me a favor."

I gave her a pair of gloves because she didn't have any. "Put these on. Let me assess him and get started with my treatment. I want you to control his C-spine so he doesn't move around a lot, and when we get to the dock we'll have the guys bring a backboard aboard."

"All right. That's fine."

"Has he been conscious at all?"

"No. He's been unconscious the whole time."

I examined the laceration on his head, which was where all the blood was coming from. Head wounds bleed a lot, so it doesn't need to be a severe injury to bleed a lot and look bad, and that was the case with this one. He had probably about a four-inch gash in his head from hitting the metal stairs when he fell. But I was still worried about his C-spine because he'd taken a good hit. Looking at the stairway, though, I could see how it might have kept him from getting too badly hurt. I put a bandage on the head wound to keep it clean and control the bleeding, and continued to assess him. Nobody seemed to know who he was. No family members were with him. I put oxygen on him, and a tourniquet, and started looking for a vein, because I was going to start an IV. It was immediately obvious that he'd had some medical issues in the past, because he had absolutely horrific veins. It was not until the third try that I finally got an IV in him; there was nothing good to shoot at.

Now he started to come around. He was a little bit groggy. I introduced myself. "I'm Bob, a paramedic from the local hospital. You're aboard a ferry. You fell. I don't want you to move, because I'm not sure if you hurt your neck when you fell. You hit your head. You've got a wound on your head."

He understood.

By this time we were almost at the dock. The ferry came in, swung around, and backed into the dock so that the cars could roll off. I got on the radio to dispatch: "Medic 14, would you advise the fire department I'm on the middle deck at the stern of the vessel. I need a backboard, collar, and the Stokes basket, because we're going to have to carry him through the ferry to get him out."

Dispatch relayed my message to the fire department, and now it was just a waiting game.

I'd put my patient on the monitor. He was fine and able to talk to me. He told me he took Dilantin for seizures. He'd felt as if he were going to have one, tried to sit down, but missed the step and knocked himself out.

The docking procedure took about five minutes. The two guys from the fire department showed up and we proceeded to backboard and collar him, put him in the Stokes basket, and carry him all the way through a couple of different decks and down off the back of the ferry into the ambulance and off to the hospital. By the time we reached the hospital, our patient was conscious and alert. There'd been no other seizure activity. For me, the experience was interesting, because I'd never boarded a vessel on a call, and had never gotten to play lights and sirens with the Coast Guard. It was fun, but it turned out to be a relatively routine call. The strange part for me was not having all of my equipment with me, not having a second pair of hands other than this nurse whom I'd never met before, and doing it on the high seas.

Things at home were not that much fun. Jen was starting to get really aggravated, and rightfully so. She was basically raising two kids all by herself all week, every week. I had a business to manage, so I ran around doing that. I'd be out on the truck and not home as much as I should have been to help her out. She was stressed out. The kids were more mobile now, so she chased them around. I wasn't there, and I wasn't being as helpful as I could or should have been. So, things were starting to get a little testy.

"Can you cut back? Can you do something? I need some help."

I was still enjoying what I was doing and being bull-headed about it, and it put a lot of strain on us.

I'd been at this for twenty-six years, and it was getting to the point where I had to start thinking about what I was going to do, whether I was going to continue. I'd thought about resigning a year or so before, but had kept on pushing through. I knew something was going to have to give soon. Maybe I could go to work every couple of weeks. But if I did that, what would my skills be like? If we didn't get a lot of calls, I'd be there putting in the hours but not treating patients and my skills would start to erode. If I cut back even further, my skills would erode further. My peers thought well of my skill set. When I got into an ambulance, they'd introduce me with the words, "This is a good medic. You'll be in good hands." Any atrophy of those skills could be dangerous to those I treated. I didn't know it at the time, but my active career as a medic was coming to a close. I did know that my priorities needed to be Jen and the boys, and the business, and maybe going out on the road as a medic wasn't part of that equation.

So, when Jen said, "You've got to cut back," I just nodded and said, "I'll think about it." It wasn't the answer she wanted to hear, but she didn't push very hard right then, so we just continued. But the career countdown timer had begun.

Thinking about that call with the Coast Guard reminded me of another one, back in 1994. I had worked an overnight shift from seven at night until seven in the morning. Freezing rain and drizzle had come down, on and off, all night long, so we raced back and forth all through the shift to motor vehicle accidents, and people who had slipped and fallen on the ice, because they hadn't been smart enough to stay home. I don't know whether freezing rain and sleet turns on people's stupid genes or what, but they don't stay home. They go out and look around. "It looks pretty on the trees, doesn't it?"

So, we'd been racing around the whole night, but by about five in the morning the weather had finally died down enough to where both the other medic and I were able to sit back, warm up a little, and try to catch a catnap.

Hopefully until the end of the shift.

I got my boots off and fell asleep for about an hour. It was a little after six in the morning when the tones went off, and I actually could not believe what I heard over the radio. "Medic 11 respond to the Coast Guard station for a fishing boat rollover."

I thought I was hearing things, because I was a little foggy. I'm used to tractor-trailer rollover, motor vehicle rollover, but not Coast

Guard and boat rollover, and not a boat rollover at six in the morning in the middle of a sleet and freezing rain storm.

I picked up the radio. "Medic 11, repeat."

"Respond to the Coast Guard station. Meet the Coast Guard for a reported boat rollover in the harbor."

I put my boots back on and started pulling on soggy clothes, grumbling. "You've got to be kidding me. Who the hell is out in this?"

When I arrived at the Coast Guard station, I was met, again, by the duty officer, who wasn't dawdling. "Grab your gear. We've got a fishing boat that rolled over in the middle of the harbor. One of the other 41s is on station with it, and we've got people trapped in the boat."

"What?"

"Just go. I'll fill you in as we go."

"Where are we going?"

He pointed. "Right there."

I could see the flashing blue light of the patrol boat about four hundred yards off to the left of the dock as we came down the gangway.

"Just be careful, man. We haven't had time to do anything with the ice." I held on to the rail. I'd got gear over my shoulder. He had the other half of my gear over his shoulder and we slid down this ramp. We didn't want to slide too far because we were liable to slide right off into the water.

Just as our feet hit the deck, the boat was ready to go, and we took off across the harbor. It was a one-minute trip. The two station's 41-footers tied up side to side.

"Go over to the other boat and we'll hand you your stuff."

So I crossed over from one boat to the next to what was now the inboard Coast Guard vessel, which was tied up alongside the rolled-over boat. Its hull faced up and the propellers were completely out of the water. To stay at the back of the boat, the Coast Guard had tied off on the propeller shaft protectors. One guy sat in the corner, shivering under a blanket.

"Who's this?" I asked.

"This is one of the deckhands."

The duty officer explained that the boat had come in with a cargo of fish in its holding tank. Like the ferries, fishing boats swung around and came into the dock stern first so it was easier to unload. But this time, the mast had accumulated a heavy coat of ice, and when the boat had made the swing, the load of fish and the tank full of water shifted. The boat was so top-heavy from all this ice and freezing rain on the super structure of the vessel that, as it turned, it flipped over. The victim in the blanket had been up on the upper deck, along with another survivor they just were pulling out of the water as we pulled alongside them.

These two had jumped overboard into the thirty-degree water. They told us, "There were two other guys that were on deck, and there are two guys below deck. We couldn't get to them. We couldn't see them. We don't know where they are."

The two guys they'd pulled out came onto our boat. They were hypothermic. I checked them quickly. "Got any injuries?"

"No, I don't have any injuries."

I got on the radio to my dispatcher. "Medic 11, respond Medic 12 to this location, and also New London's two ambulances. We have two hypothermic victims coming in with the Coast Guard, and there are four other victims at this point unaccounted for. I'll be on scene for the foreseeable future and notify the supervisors what's going on."

The Coast Guard vessel that brought me out left with the two crewmen. There was nothing I could do for them. They weren't injured. They were just cold. They were going to go to the hospital to get checked out, because they hadn't been in the water all that long. I had the other medic standing by at the Coast Guard station. My thinking at that moment was that these other four guys were going to come out really quickly. They were going to be hypothermic. They might be cut, bruised, whatever. I was going to load them onto the second Coast Guard vessel, and ship them to shore to the other medic, sort of a survivor ferry service. He could take them to the hospital, and come back.

The other two, who'd been on deck, were found fairly quickly. One guy had swum to shore, and the cops told us that he'd called in and he was safe. So, now three were left unaccounted for. Another guy was fished out after swimming up to the Coast Guard boat. We had four. He wasn't hurt.

"Where are the other two?" I asked.

"They're below deck. They can't get out."

"What do you mean 'they can't get out'?"

He said, "There's no way to get to them."

We were standing out on the deck of the Coast Guard boat. I'd never been this cold in my life. My teeth were chattering. I had a uniform shirt and a raincoat, because I had been in and out of the truck all night long. I was not prepared to be out for prolonged periods of time in this weather.

The cabins on the Coast Guard boats are so small that only a couple of people can fit in there at a time. Everybody else has to be out on deck.

There was one crewman with the Coast Guard whose job was to keep chipping ice, because the ice from the freezing rain was building up on the deck and the rails of the boat and everything else as fast as he could chip it off. I had a life jacket, which I was thankful for, because I was at least was a little bit warmer. Suddenly, as we were standing there, we heard banging.

Everybody stopped. "Shut up. Shut up. Shut up. What's that?"

The banging continued, and we realized it was coming from inside the hull of the overturned ship.

The guy in charge of the Coast Guard boat, the coxswain, asked, "Where is that coming from?"

We tried to pinpoint where it was coming from and found it was from the middle area of the boat. We hadn't ferried the last deckhand back to shore yet. "What's there?" we asked.

"Well, there's the wheelhouse. It's middle forward and then there's the openings to the holds where the fish are, and the lower deck ladders are towards the aft of the boat."

About this time we saw another boat coming across from the Coast Guard station. They'd brought a third vessel out with divers from the fire department. They'd also called for divers from the Navy submarine base, which was about a mile up the river from our location.

We all felt a little bit better as the two fire department divers came aboard our boat. They were going to dive in, free the two guys, and this would be over.

We were told that the additional Navy divers would arrive in about ten minutes so we would have four divers on the scene. I was just waiting for something to do and trying to stay out of everybody's way. I knew one of the divers from the fire department. His name was Dave. He got ready, was attached to a safety rope, and went in the water. He was back up in less than two minutes.

"There's no way I'm getting in there."

"What's going on?"

"The fishing nets have flipped over, and we're going to have to cut our way through the fishing nets to get in there."

He was looking for knives. He was looking for whatever he could use to get in there. He found a big diving knife and dropped back into the water. He went in for a few minutes at a time as he tried to cut through the nets and get to the men. We could still hear the hammering, but it was getting fainter.

This is not good. They're in frigid water. We don't know whether they're in an airtight compartment. We don't know anything about where they are. This is not going to turn out well if we don't hurry up.

The Navy divers arrived. Now there were four of them going in, two at a time. They kept trying over and over again. They went in for five or ten minutes, came back up, went down for another five or ten minutes, came back up. Because the water was so cold, their hands froze up. They couldn't operate the knife to cut and pull the heavy netting, and there was no other way to get in. We'd been on scene forty-five minutes now. The hammering was getting softer and softer, and then it stopped.

Crap.

We couldn't get to them. We couldn't get through the steel hull. Unless something really dramatic happened, there was nothing that we could do to save those two guys.

It was probably one of the most helpless feelings I've ever had. We had every possible resource on scene in less than fifteen minutes after it happened, and nobody could do anything. It was just horrendous to stand there knowing what they were going through under water because of our own experiences with the freezing weather above the water.

The rescue went on and on, and it got to a point where it was very obvious that there was nothing we were going to be able to do. I asked the Coast Guard, "Do me a favor. Can you take me and my gear in? We're going to do a crew change."

I passed the report on to my relief, a medic named John. "They're not going to be able to get these two guys out. Dave's been in; the Navy divers have been in. Nobody can get in there to get at these guys. When we first started they were hammering like crazy, and now we haven't heard anything for ninety minutes." The call was now more than two hours old. The Coast Guard was in recovery mode. John came out and stood vigil. He told me afterward that the state police dive recovery team responded and cut a hole in the hull. But it took several hours for them to finally be able to get in and find the guys. Hypothermia had taken them. Just standing out there on the deck of the Coast Guard boat, I had honestly never felt that cold, that pissed off, and that helpless in my career.

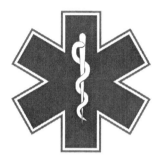

CHAPTER 26

COP VS. DEER VS. WROUGHT IRON FENCE

COP VS. DEER VS. WROUGHT IRON FENCE

During the last ten years of my career, I was an EMT instructor, taking people who had no EMS background at all and turning them into basic EMTs. I also assisted with a couple of paramedic classes, taking people who were EMTs and teaching them how to become paramedics. For more than fifteen years I had been a field training officer, or a preceptor, as they're called. I would be assigned paramedic students and bring them out on calls, just as I myself had gone on calls in the '80s, except I wasn't as nasty to them as my instructor was, and I didn't turn the drug box upside-down as my instructor had done to me. But I did make them go through the box and memorize what went in there.

We'd run scenarios as we were going to calls. I'd say, "Okay. We're going to a chest pain call. Tell me what you're thinking. Tell me what you're planning to do."

It's the preceptor's job to get the kids, as we call them, ready to work beside us. It is something every preceptor takes very seriously, because preceptors are the last bit of training the students have. Their job is to tie all of the students' learning together, everything the students have done in the hospital, everything they've done in the simulator labs, and everything that they've studied in their books.

We had six or eight weeks to take all of that learning and make sure that they could apply it to actual patients.

Students' clinical training time in the hospital is fairly controlled. It's not at all controlled in the back of the ambulance or on scenes. You're looking to see that the new medics know what they're doing, that they can take charge of a scene that's chaotic, that they can lead the team of people to take care of the patient, and that they can think on their feet and get things done. When things don't go perfectly, can they adapt quickly enough? Every student comes to the trucks expecting that a heart attack is going to look like this, and a diabetic situation is going to look like that, and a car accident is going to look like the pictures in their books. It becomes very clear, very quickly, that patients don't read the book. Cars are upside-down. Patients have diabetic issues, which trigger heart complications too. They have a seizure, but they have it on a ferry and fall down a flight of stairs and crack their head. The street is different, so we have to evaluate their readiness.

I've always loved having the students with me. Not that I'm necessarily the best paramedic in the world; I think I'm a good paramedic, and I think I'm good with people. But I want the ability to train those folks, because they're the ones who could be taking care of me or my family. I take it as a serious responsibility.

At home, things were definitely coming to a head. On both of the previous two Fridays, instead of working noon to midnight, I had gotten home really late. Just because the shift was supposed to end at a certain time never meant that it would. The previous Friday, the shift ended with a call in which a police cruiser was struck by a drunk driver. We had to have the fire department extricate the officer from the cruiser, and his condition was serious enough for us to call the helicopter. We ended up landing a Lifestar chopper in the middle of an icy parking lot, because it was the only nearby place we could put the chopper down.

It's an interesting experience to have a 120-mile-an-hour rotor wash on an icy surface, as you're trying to get to the helicopter, load the patient, and not kill yourself by sliding into the tail rotor.

The guy in the other car had bounced off the cruiser, rolled his car over a couple of times, and broken his neck.

I had to presume him dead while the firefighters were cutting the cruiser apart. It was obvious that he was dead, his body was facing forward, but his head was looking backward over his shoulder, ironically in the direction of the cruiser. So, I'd arrived home at four in the morning. I got no sympathy from Jen because at six in the morning the kids needed to be fed, and Jen needed a break. I got two hours of sleep, and she woke me, saying, "You need to help me with the kids," and rightfully so. I was exhausted and I knew that I was going to have to make some serious decisions fairly soon.

But I didn't know when I went out the following Friday that it was going to be my last shift. I had a young female medic student, Lindsay, working with me. She told me gleefully that she was only nineteen. My response was, "You realize I've been in EMS twenty-six years and you're only nineteen?"

I was feeling very old at this point, and the fact that she was getting such a kick out of rubbing it in wasn't helping. Finally I just muttered, "Kids should be seen and not heard, so you just sit in the back of the truck and be quiet."

It was about eleven at night, one hour to go, and we were toned out for a police officer with an unknown injury. I knew this was going to be an interesting call, because any time the cops didn't want to say exactly what was going on, there was a reason.

We responded to an address in the area of Broad and Jefferson streets. I knew the only thing in the area of that particular intersection was a cemetery. On one side of the street there was a chain link fence about four feet high, and on the other side, the older cemetery had a six-foot, wrought iron fence that was about five hundred yards long. We were right down the street, so we were going to beat the ambulance to the scene, because the ambulance had to come from the other side of town. As we rolled up to the scene, we saw cops everywhere. Something wasn't right. "Lindsay, I'm not sure what this is going to be, but just stick with me, because something's strange."

As we pulled up and stopped, I could see a cop on the fence, hanging onto it. A whole bunch of cops were around him. I figured maybe he'd broken his ankle, or his foot was caught, or something like that. I looked again, and to the left of this bunch of cops was a deer, and this deer was also stuck on this fence, impaled on it. I just looked at everybody in the truck. "I have no words for this."

We stopped right by the action and started to get out of the truck, but all the cops were screaming, "Don't stop there! Pull up, pull up, pull up."

"What?"

"Get in the truck and pull up."

They all pointed farther up the street.

As I closed the door and started to pull the truck away, I heard gunshots. They had to shoot the deer, and they didn't want us around, because the way they were shooting, if the bullet had gone through the deer and hit the concrete sidewalk, it could have ricocheted into the truck. Okay. So, we pulled up, got out, grabbed the gear, and approached the group of officers.

"What the hell is going on?"

The cops explained. "The deer got caught on the fence, and Jimmy tried to help him. Now he's impaled on the fence."

The deer apparently had tried to hop the fence, didn't make it, and was impaled on the fence. The cop was on patrol, saw the deer, and tried to hop over the fence, because he figured he could get to the other side without having to go all the way through the cemetery. The deer heard him coming, got scared, and started thrashing. Jimmy lost his balance and ended up with a wrought iron rail through his thigh. Now, the deer's on the fence rocking the fence because he's trying to get off, and the cop has the wrought iron rail of the fence impaled in his leg, and he can't get off either. They had to shoot the deer to stop it from shaking the fence. Now, we had to figure out how we were going to get this guy down. We couldn't lift him off, because you don't take impaled objects out. You bandage around them and let the surgeon do the removal.

The cop was in a lot of pain, begging. "Give me something. Give me something for the pain."

I said, "I can't even get to you."

The other cops were holding him up so he didn't slip down any farther, because he was tired. He'd been on the fence for ten minutes. My trainee, Lindsay, was probably all of a hundred pounds. "Hey, guys. Without impaling Lindsay on the fence, we need to put her on the other side of the fence so she can treat Jimmy."

"Okay."

So three guys carefully hoisted my hundred-pound paramedic student up over the fence.

I asked her, "Can you get at his arm?"

"Yeah."

"Start an IV."

I handed her all the stuff through the fence and she started an IV.

"You got any allergies?" I asked my patient.

"No."

"Take any meds?"

"No."

"Any medical issues?"

"Yeah, I've got a freaking fence in my leg."

"So I see. Besides that?"

"No."

I handed Lindsay the morphine. "Give him two milligrams of morphine through the IV."

"Aren't you going to call for orders?" she asked me.

"Just give him two milligrams of morphine. It's on me. I'll take responsibility for it. I'll tell the docs later. I can't go to the truck, call the hospital to ask, and supervise you at the same time, and he needs the morphine. Give him the morphine."

She was nervous. "But, but..."

"Listen to me. Give him the morphine. I can't reach him. You can. Draw it up." I held the flashlight so she could see how much she was drawing into the syringe. She held it up for me to confirm the dosage and then gave him the medication. It didn't do anything.

The fire department arrived, and we discussed how to extricate him. Lindsay was still on the other side of the fence, taking the cop's vital signs, trying to talk to him. He was still in agony, moaning, "It's not touching it!"

"Lindsay, give him two more."

"But..."

"Give him two more milligrams of morphine!"

She did. It took the edge off, and he was okay for the moment.

The guys were trying to figure out what to do, because they had to cut the fence, but if they used the big saw, it would make the fence vibrate like crazy. That's not good when the fence is impaled in your leg. One of the guys brought out a ratchet and started unbolting one section of the fence, and the other guys brought the cutters. The firefighter said to me, "Listen, we've figured a way to cut this without vibrating it, but he's going to end up with a three-foot piece of fence sticking out of his leg when we're done."

I replied, "That's okay. We'll package him the way he is and take him to the hospital. It's a big ambulance. We'll make it work."

Lindsay gives him another two milligrams of morphine. But now the problem was he was starting to feel really comfortable, starting to relax a little bit. The guys held him up because now he had six milligrams of morphine on board, and he was feeling pretty damn good.

They told him, "Stop moving around."

The firefighters cut the fence and we actually ended up with about a two-foot chunk of wrought iron fence sticking out of his leg. We positioned it so it didn't move much. We put him in the ambulance backward, because it was the only way we could get him and the fence and the stretcher in. There were four of us in the ambulance. Before we left, I asked the sergeant, "Could you take his gun? I don't want his gun in the ambulance while he is under the influence of morphine."

A cop is trained to instinctively protect himself if somebody reaches for his gun. So, one cop had to hold each of his hands. The sergeant stood in front of him. "Jimmy, we're going to take your gun belt off. Don't mess around," he said so Jimmy knew what was going on.

Now, our hospital was five minutes away, but this was a trauma call. We had an impaled object. I didn't know exactly how close the rail was to the femoral artery in his leg, because I didn't have X-rays, but I wasn't taking a chance, so I called it in as a trauma alert to the other hospital, which is a fifteen-minute ride.

"Jimmy," I said, "I'm sorry we've got to do this, but protocol says it's trauma. We've got to take you to the trauma center. It's a longer ride, but I've got no choice."

He was on oxygen and not feeling a lot of pain. I'd never driven to the hospital with a cop under the influence of morphine and with two feet of wrought iron fence sticking out of him. I told Lindsay, "Well, at least you're going to have the most interesting paramedic student story of the week."

Lindsay just shook her head. "Nobody's going to believe me."

We pulled into the hospital, the surgeon looked at us, and said, "What the hell is this?"

"This is the officer with a fence in his leg near his femoral artery that we called about."

"Why'd you call a trauma alert for this?"

"I don't know. It met the criteria for me. He's got an impaled object near his femoral artery."

"It's nowhere near his femoral artery."

"Okay. I'm saying it is," I said. "You're saying it's not. When he's your patient, you do what you want with him. But regardless, he's a cop, and we take care of our own. So, better to be a little overly cautious and make sure everybody's here in case something happens. Better safe than sorry."

The surgeon just snorted. "This does not meet the trauma guidelines. This is ridiculous."

I'd been at this for twenty-six years. I was working part-time, so if I lost my medic job I really didn't care because I had my business. This doctor was just being a pompous ass, in my humble opinion, so

I said rather loudly, "Are you for real?" A collective hush fell over the trauma room.

The doctor turned around. "What'd you say?"

"I said, are you for real? I call a trauma alert, because I've got a cop with an impaled object, and number one, we should take care of our own. But number two, it met the criteria, and you're giving me a hard time about this?"

"This is not a trauma alert. This is ridiculous. I shouldn't be here."

Now he's pissed me off.

"You shouldn't be here for a number of reasons, the least of which is a trauma. I don't know what kind of a doctor you are, we've never met, but you're an idiot."

The nurses looked at each other. He came over and got right in my face, "What is your name?"

I gave it to him and kept going. "You and I can talk about this later if you'd like, or we can talk about it now. But I'm going to go write my run report. You have a patient to take care of. I'm leaving." And I walked out.

One of the nurses followed me outside. "We've always wanted somebody to say that to him. But it's going to get ugly."

"It can get ugly if it wants. I really don't care. We did what was in the best interest of the patient."

"I would have called a trauma alert too."

"I appreciate that."

We went into the EMS office to write up the paperwork and then we put the truck back together. I signed all of Lindsay's paperwork so she officially had her paramedic intern story for class. The fact that she gave morphine was a big deal for a paramedic student, because it doesn't happen all that often. Usually the medic wants to give it, not the medic student.

I see her from time to time, and she always talks about it. "You and the fence. I can't believe you called the doctor an idiot."

She still works as a medic, and by all accounts is a very good one.

I'm proud to have had a small hand in helping a number of students over the years become EMTs and paramedics. What they became, they became on their own, but I like to think that I taught them well along the way.

This was Friday night, so on Monday morning I sent an e-mail to my boss at the hospital and told him what had happened and what I had said. I knew the EMS coordinator at the other hospital personally, so I called him myself. "Happy Monday."

"Uh-huh."

"I assume you heard about Friday."

"Uh-huh."

"Is it going to go any farther than this? Do you need an incident report from me? Do you need me to come and meet with him?"

"No. No. But are you coming back anytime soon?"

"No."

"That's good. Between you, me and the lamppost, I'm glad you said it. Between you and me as EMS coordinator, thanks a hell of a lot."

"Well, you know, if I'm going to go out, I might as well go out on a high note."

That night I got home at four forty-five in the morning. That made two Friday nights in a row I'd come in late: one was four; one was four forty-five in the morning. Jen looked at me and shook her head at six in the morning as we fed the kids. She didn't mince words. "You've got to make a choice. We can't keep doing this."

"You're right. I'm done. I'll go out on that note."

Later that week I gave my notice to the hospital and said I was resigning as an active paramedic. In my letter I said that it was more important for me to go out at the top of my game, having done a good job, than for me to work less and less and less, and risk having my skills degrade to the point at which I might do some damage and hurt somebody. I'd rather have the legacy, "Hey, Bob was a pretty good medic," than, "Bob should have retired a long time ago, before he hurt that kid."

It was the right thing to do, for all the right reasons, but it was a very difficult step to take. For twenty-six years the job had defined me, consumed me, if you will, and now, overnight I'd gone from "I'm a paramedic" to "I'm just a business owner who *used to be* a paramedic."

I kept my license, and decided that I would work at the hospital as a volunteer driver on the medic truck when time permitted.

For the next couple of years I worked once a month with another paramedic. The medic on the truck was the primary, and I was the volunteer driver. Since I was also a paramedic, we had the ability to bounce stuff off each other, but I was not responsible for the patient. The other medic was.

I spent time building my business. I had twenty-three people working for my company. I also found that it was a lot more rewarding for me to be home with Jen and the boys, to work a normal schedule, and be home at night. I traveled as needed, but not as much as I used to. I wanted to be at my kids' baseball games and school events.

When the kids were first born, I started taking Tuesdays off. Boys' Day, we called it. I'd hang with the twins and give Jen a break.

That continued for ten years. When the kids were little, Jen would go to the office and I would take care of the boys. Now that the kids are in school, Jen and I take every Tuesday off so that we can have some time together.

When they were infants, I'd go run errands with them. Hey, if I could manage a scene with critically injured patients, I could manage two kids who needed a bottle and a diaper. I'd put them in the stroller, and I'd go to the mall or do whatever I needed to do. Mothers would look at me as if I were from Mars. One woman actually came up to me when I was at the mall. I was having a sandwich and feeding the twins, and she walked up and asked, "Do you need any help?"

"I appreciate it, but I'm good."

"Are you by yourself?"

"Yes. My wife's at work."

"I wouldn't let my husband have the kids by himself in the living room."

"Well, I'm offering training classes. If you want to send him over, I'll teach him how to do it."

"No. No, no, no," she said as she slowly backed away.

As the kids got older, on Tuesdays we would go to the aquarium and the Science Center. We would go down to Battleship Cove in Massachusetts and climb through gun turrets. When the kids are on vacation now, so am I. We bought a beach house in Wells, Maine, six years ago, and in the summertime when the kids are off, I commute back and forth to Connecticut. I work for three days, take some work with me, and go back and forth to Maine all summer. I put in three fourteen-hour days. I used to work twelve-hour shifts on the ambulance, so what's fourteen hours in the office?

I can honestly say from time to time I miss the work. Actually I miss interacting with patients. I still stop at the scenes of accidents when I'm driving by. As a matter of fact, I stopped at one in my neighborhood just the other day. I was putting stuff in the truck to head home from Maine, and I heard screech, bang, thud, "ugh," on the road that runs right behind my house. I immediately grabbed my equipment and went running, because I thought a kid had been hit by a car. There were a lot of people out, lots of pedestrian traffic on that street, and people didn't drive as slowly as they should have.

About four houses down from my house, I found a young lady who had lost control of her moped. She had hit a parked car, bounced onto the street, and rolled three or four times into my neighbor's yard. The guy riding with her was an off-duty firefighter from New Hampshire. Fortunately she wasn't badly hurt, a lot of road rash, some fairly deep gashes in her toes and ankle and knee, and a completely ruined pedicure. We kept her calm until the Wells police, fire, and ambulance arrived, and they did a great job. I have to be honest, it felt good to be back in that situation and to be in control.

All my neighbors were there. They knew that I did something with ambulances, but they didn't really know what, and we hadn't really talked much about it. Then, out of nowhere I came down the street and took over. What can I say? Old habits—they really do die hard.

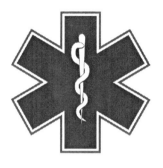

CHAPTER 27

THE EMS SYSTEM IN CHAOS

THE EMS SYSTEM IN CHAOS

I opened my own consulting practice in March 1988. My first clients were agencies I already knew and had interacted with through the hospital. I did lots of CPR training, EMT training, and paramedic training. I had set up disaster drills at the Navy base and the nuclear plant. More and more, I found that clients would come to me with requests for different kinds of assistance. "Can you help us with filing paperwork for the state?"

Yeah, I knew how to do that, been doing it for years. So I'd offer that service. Then somebody said, "Can you help us with billing?" So I started a billing company, which was the first, and is now the largest EMS billing service serving CT ambulance companies. We handle about 30 percent of the ambulance services in Connecticut.

Every time clients would come in asking for help with some aspect of EMS operations, management, or leadership, we found a way to help them. We always found a resource that we could bring to the table, and our business grew and grew and grew. Now, twenty-five years later, we're arguably one of the top five EMS leadership firms in the country.

Having been around for such a long time and having worked with hundreds of clients, I find myself responding to a new kind of chaos: the chaos of a misunderstood system.

The general public and the politicians really don't know what EMS is capable of, what we're supposed to do, how we should be funded, or how we should be staffed. We have dwindling numbers of people coming into the industry in many states. But we still have lots of dedicated paid and volunteer EMS professionals out there doing their jobs and giving up their family time as I had.

The system itself is in chaos. America's 9-1-1 system is hanging by a thread. Many agencies are living Medicare check to Medicaid check. A number of agencies have had to eliminate positions, cut back benefits, and put fewer trucks on the road, even as the system demands are increasing. Our office is getting phone calls on a weekly basis from all around the country, from service chiefs and municipal officials trying to figure out how to properly equip their communities for 9-1-1 calls, how to serve the patients.

As I write this book, the Patient Protection and Affordable Care Act, otherwise known as Obamacare is looming and expected to impact the EMS industry hard beginning in 2014. It's clear to me that the system has a very real potential to collapse.

I wrote an article recently for *EMS World* in which I predicted that 20 percent of the ambulance services in this country aren't going to be around in 2020. You can read it on my blog @ www.Holdsworth.com/blog. They're going to be acquired, merged, or simply go out of business, because of problems with either money or staffing. Nobody seems to want to take on the challenge of fixing that. The other part of the problem is a leadership deficit; nobody wants to take on the job of leading these organizations, partly because of the time commitment and partly because there's really no formalized chain of training and career path for people to follow.

Post 9/11, the EMS system is expected to do more and do it with less. Homeland Security issues, more responses to mysterious white powder calls, an increase in ambulance standbys for hazardous materials incidents, the need for additional training and additional supplies that need to be carried are all added demands on an already overtaxed system. Most counties or bigger communities have started to build caches of disaster supplies in case they're the next target. EMS is supposed to be able to deal with that too. So many agencies out there are expected to keep their fingers on the pulse of EMS, but the reality is that they're not working together. The federal government agencies are not working in collaboration with state and regional organizations. Internally there are arguments between fire-based EMS, private for-profit companies, nonprofit stand alone EMS agencies, and hospital-based EMS. Most of these issues revolve around turf and dollars.

That's the kind of chaos my business colleagues and I are routinely called upon to try and resolve. I jokingly said that our company logo should be a striped shirt and a whistle, because we're pulled into these disputes and taxed with solving them; doing studies of EMS systems, running budget scenarios, looking for ways to recruit and retain people and train the next generation of leaders.

The system is in chaos, and as revenue continues to shrink and more people begin to use the 9-1-1 ambulance systems as the health-care safety net, it will get worse. None of these problems can be solved without strong leadership.

In order to help address the leadership vacuum in the industry, we've established the EMS Leadership Institute (**www.WeLeadEMS.com**). We offer online learning courses where both future leaders and existing leaders, can get state-of-the-art education and training to help them run their organizations more efficiently. We're bringing in industry leaders from across the spectrum of ambulance, fire, health, and the business communities.

My observation is that this cross-pollination is necessary because one of the things we're not good at as an industry is looking outside the EMS box. We don't look to other types of businesses for opportunities or ideas. My background, both in EMS and in other industries, has given me a perspective on how things work in other industries, which I plan to bring to EMS. Not a lot of people have that ability.

At both the beginning and the end of the book, you'll find a page that offers you an opportunity to test out the EMS Leadership Institute for yourself. Try it and see whether this resource for learning is something that can help you become a better leader, help you run your system better, and help you in dealing with your own kind of chaos.

OUTRO

As I was looking back, digging into the memory banks and my files for the stories I've shared with you in these pages, I found myself making one of those old-fashioned Ben Franklin pros and cons lists.

A full range of emotions came back to me as I committed these stories to paper. I remembered the sights and the sounds, the frustrations, the families in anger or anguish or disbelief, the joy we felt in saving a life or mitigating a tragedy, and the helplessness we felt when that wasn't possible. I tried to choose the best from the more than 20,000 patient interactions I've had to illustrate the highs, lows, and the stresses felt by all in EMS.

I had some time to look back at all the things that I've gotten from thirty-three years in this industry. They went in the pro column. I also looked at all the things that left scars. It actually worked out to be pretty even between the two sides of the ledger.

On the pro side of the list were the valued thirty-year-plus friendships created and maintained with many of the people who've appeared in these stories, and others that will be acknowledged at the end of the book. In my role as an agency leader, EMS coordinator, and business owner, I've had a hand in creating hundreds of jobs for EMS professionals throughout the years. I've had the ability to impact hundreds of thousands of patients, and have personally treated close to 20,000 patients, by my best estimate, which gives me a tremendous sense of satisfaction.

I would not have met my wife and best friend, Jennifer, had I not taken the entrepreneurial path and opened my business, which means I would not have had the two best gifts I never thought I wanted, my two sons. I wouldn't have been a dad. I would probably have still been working too many hours, running though a series of broken relationships, and been on a much more self-destructive path. Jennifer and the boys, those three reasons alone make the thirty-three years rewarding.

By most people's definition, I have been successful in a business dedicated to helping others. I've been able to have a positive impact on various regions around the country and a fairly significant impact on sections of the state of Connecticut, by providing paramedics for the first time and improving the service. In my mind that means that I've helped build and create a legacy, because those agencies continue to serve people every day. I'm proud to have had a hand in crafting them, building them, or making them better in someway. Those are all the good things that have come out of my years in the business.

However, along the way, I, in common with other EMS professionals around the country, have sacrificed irreplaceable hours of family time, missed family events, and strained friendships and marriages, in some cases to their breaking point.

Because of all the time I spent on the truck, I've struggled until very recently with a lack of emotional connection and real intimacy in relationships. Everything was compartmentalized and it was too easy to turn off and discard a piece of a relationship or the whole relationship in many cases. I've got a long, sorry history of failed relationships, a failed first marriage, and an almost-failed second marriage, thanks to important things I left undone as well as things I did that I should not have done. To her credit, Jen stayed, and we are probably in a better place than we've ever been in fifteen years of marriage. I owe her a lot for her courage in sticking with me.

On the physical side, there are still sights, sounds, and smells that will bring back memories of calls from years ago. I've had several EMS-related injuries of my own, from being involved in a high speed ambulance crash, being stabbed by a patient, and having injured my back on several occasions to the point where, between the ambulance accident and carrying patients in weird positions for years, if I don't get up every morning and stretch, I end up with a headache because of the damage that was done.

When you balance those things one against the other, some people would ask, "Was it all worth it?" To my way of thinking, all of the good things in my life have come as a result of friendships, partnerships, and the good side of the business—and yes, those good things greatly overshadow the losses.

I'm grateful, proud and happy that finally my life, both personal and professional, is now in a really good place, and that there's a whole lot less chaos thirty-three years later. It's critically important to remember that **Wading into Chaos is what we do, it's not how we have to live our lives.**

I can only wish you the good fortune to realize what's important sooner in your life than I did. Life's too short, enjoy it!

ACKNOWLEDGMENTS

I firmly believe that each of us is a compilation and a reflection of all of the people we've come into close contact with throughout life, which in my case is family, friends, the more than twenty thousand patients I've treated, and several thousand coworkers and clients. Their reflections leave both positive and negative impressions since every interaction is either a lesson that includes something good that you can emulate, or something bad that is a lesson in what not to do. Either way, learning happens. I have been blessed with many people in my life who have provided me with more good lessons than bad.

I want to take a few words to say thanks to them in the order in which they appeared in my life:

- To my parents, Bob and Anne, who said no, then allowed me to creatively get what I wanted anyway; who taught me the lessons of working hard for what I wanted; who gave me everything I *needed* and taught me how to get the things I *wanted*. They always supported me even if they didn't agree with me, like when my mother objected to my four years working as a prison guard. I cannot thank them enough for the sacrifices they made to provide a great home and a tight-knit family, and for allowing me to get the best education a C student could have. Thank you!

- To Marty Walsh, my grandfather, who also taught me how to think creatively to get what I wanted, especially after my parents had said no. He also showed me that enjoyable work was a good thing. He worked well into his seventies and was well respected as a craftsman in the jewelry industry in Boston. He always spoke his mind, and he had lots of friends in spite of that. A very important lesson for all of us.

- To my Aunt Mary who taught me that any subject should be fair game for discussion, and that there is good in almost everything and everyone if you look for it. She also taught me that you could almost always find the good over a cup of tea and some blunt conversation. I miss our conversations.

- To my siblings, Ellen, Paul, and Susan, who have always been there when I needed to talk, vent, or just have fun together. I am fortunate that my folks raised us to actually like each other. On his eightieth birthday, my dad said, "I'm proud that you all keep in touch and turned out to be good kids." So am I.

- To Mark, Jim, Blair, Bruce, Bob, Greg, Jeff, Todd, Cody, Glenn, and all of the other "convicts" who proclaim themselves to be my friends. It's not an easy task but some of them are still there after more than thirty-five years and have taught me that I can't ever take myself too seriously. They know the truth.

- To Richard Meny, a businessman who also didn't know how to take no for an answer and who, many years ago, trusted a twenty-six-year-old kid to run his multimillion dollar business solely on his instinct that I'd "do okay." Rest peacefully, Dick.

- To my partners, students, and colleagues: It has been a privilege to have worked alongside you, often under very trying and stressful conditions. I've been fortunate to witness your professionalism, courage, intelligence, and humor, and I thank you all for doing what you do.

- To my business partner, Tim. We have been friends and worked together, helping others for a lot of years, and we shared slightly different career paths which finally crossed once and for all into a business partnership in 1997. Thanks for your friendship, your business ethics, your stories, and for making me laugh along the way—oh yeah, and for buying into the company when you did. We bought a great house with the money.

- To my beautiful and intelligent wife, Jennifer, for putting up with my moods and the various "new ideas" that I constantly come up with. It was my desire to spend more time with her and eventually retire to a small house near the beach that led me to change the way I worked and realize that time off is important. She also gave me the two best gifts I never thought I wanted.

- To my twin boys, Jack and Chris, who've taught me a lot about myself, made me look at things like a two-year-old again, and constantly ask the question: "B'cuz why?" I've found that the answers to that question spark the biggest changes.

- To my editor, Jenny Tripp, and Alison Morse, Brooke White, Kim Hall, Denis Boyles, and Adam Witty, the team at Advantage Media, who believed in me enough to take on this project, which was outside their comfort zone.

- Lastly, my thanks to you, since, by purchasing this book, you have now entered my life. I look forward to your feedback after you've gone through the words in this book, and I hope that the stories capture your imagination and inspire you to serve others in some way.

Drop me an email at bob@WadingIntoChaos.com, or join me on Twitter and Facebook.

To read additional stories, discuss booking me as a speaker for your event or conference, or to stock up on the latest *Wading into Chaos* gear, visit **www.WadingIntoChaos.com.**

READ THIS PAGE **ONLY** IF YOU ARE IN EMS or FIRE:

MOST RIDICULOUS

OFFER **EVER**

A message from the author
Bob Holdsworth:

I want to offer you something that I'm not giving to ANYONE else in the industry. Whether you're a Chief of Service, a brand new supervisor, or are new to the field and have aspirations of EMS leadership, I'm giving you a two-month **FREE subscription** to the EMS Leadership Institute.

My team and I built the institute specifically for people like you, providing insightful topic experts, marketing swipe files, monthly webinars, and the game-changing resources that will boost your leadership to a new level.

Claim your **COMPLIMENTARY** two-month membership TODAY and I'll also send you a BONUS gift...

www.WeLeadEMS.com
Use coupon code: CHAOS

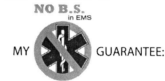

MY GUARANTEE:

Join the EMS Leadership Institute, use it for two months, FREE and get my special bonus gift.

If you think it **SUCKS** and you're not happy with it, I'll cancel your account and refund the money you paid for this book just for wasting your time.

Log on to **WeLeadEMS.com** and use coupon code: **CHAOS**

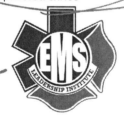

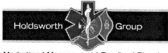

Marketing I Management I Funding I Planning

National Experience. Local Solutions.℠

Need instant assistance with your EMS or Fire Department? My team has over 70-combined years of experience in the EMS consulting industry, offering unique, tailored solutions for YOUR service. Log on to www.Holdsworth.com to learn more. **When people need help - they call EMS. When EMS needs help - they call us!**

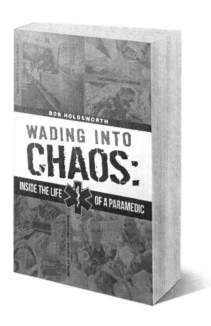

How can you use this book?

MOTIVATE

EDUCATE

THANK

INSPIRE

PROMOTE

CONNECT

Why have a custom version of *Wading into Chaos*?

- Build personal bonds with customers, prospects, employees, donors, and key constituencies

- Develop a long-lasting reminder of your event, milestone, or celebration

- Provide a keepsake that inspires change in behavior and change in lives

- Deliver the ultimate "thank you" gift that remains on coffee tables and bookshelves

- Generate the "wow" factor

Books are thoughtful gifts that provide a genuine sentiment that other promotional items cannot express. They promote employee discussions and interaction, reinforce an event's meaning or location, and they make a lasting impression. Use your book to say "Thank You" and show people that you care.

Wading into Chaos is available in bulk quantities and in customized versions at special discounts for corporate, institutional, and educational purposes. To learn more please contact our Special Sales team at:

1.866.775.1696 • sales@advantageww.com • www.AdvantageSpecialSales.com

CPSIA information can be obtained at www.ICGtesting.com
Printed in the USA
BVOW011427230113

311415BV00012B/266/P